Schizophrenia

O P L
OXFORD PSYCHIATRY LIBRARY

Schizophrenia

Revised Edition

Professor David J. Castle

Chair of Psychiatry, St Vincent's Hospital,
The University of Melbourne,
Victoria, Australia

Professor Peter F. Buckley

Professor and Chairman,
Department of Psychiatry,
Associate Dean for Leadership Development,
Medical College of Georgia,
Augusta, USA

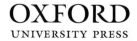

OXFORD
UNIVERSITY PRESS

OXFORD
UNIVERSITY PRESS

Great Clarendon Street, Oxford OX2 6DP

Oxford University Press is a department of the University of Oxford.
It furthers the University's objective of excellence in research, scholarship,
and education by publishing worldwide in

Oxford New York

Auckland Cape Town Dar es Salaam Hong Kong Karachi
Kuala Lumpur Madrid Melbourne Mexico City Nairobi
New Delhi Shanghai Taipei Toronto

With offices in

Argentina Austria Brazil Chile Czech Republic France Greece
Guatemala Hungary Italy Japan Poland Portugal Singapore
South Korea Switzerland Thailand Turkey Ukraine Vietnam

Oxford is a registered trade mark of Oxford University Press
in the UK and in certain other countries

Published in the United States
by Oxford University Press Inc., New York

First published 2008
Revised edition published 2011

British Library Cataloguing in Publication Data
Data available

Library of Congress Cataloging in Publication Data
Data available

Typeset by Newgen Imaging Systems (P) Ltd., Chennai, India
Printed in China
on acid-free paper through
Asia Pacific Offset

ISBN 978–0–19–969303–0

10 9 8 7 6 5 4 3 2 1

Whilst every effort has been made to ensure that the contents of this book are as
complete, accurate and up-to-date as possible at the date of writing, Oxford
University Press is not able to give any guarantee or assurance that such is the case.
Readers are urged to take appropriately qualified medical advice in all cases. The
information in this book is intended to be useful to the general reader, but should
not be used as a means of self-diagnosis or for the prescription of medication.

Contents

Foreword

This slim volume will be a welcome addition to the shelves of anyone in the mental health field. It provides a succinct and up-to-date overview of schizophrenia using a question-and-answer format. This makes it easily accessible and a ready quick reference guide. It is clearly written, and not just presents the received wisdom but also tackles some of the more controversial issues pertinent to schizophrenia in a balanced manner.

Part 1 addresses classification, clinical features, epidemiology, aetiological factors, brain abnormalities, and neurochemistry; Part 2 turns to management, covering service models, and biological, psychological, and social aspects of treatment. The text is liberally augmented with tables, figures, and fact boxes, enhancing the ease of reading.

Part 3 is a stand-alone section of patient/carer information regarding medications used in psychiatry, tips about dealing with side effects and enhancing adherence, and information about looking after physical health. This section will be particularly useful for clinicians who wish to provide their patients with materials which are balanced and 'user friendly'.

Drs Castle and Buckley are well recognized for their research and teaching regarding schizophrenia. Their joint experience spans the United Kingdom, Ireland, the United States, and Australia and gives the book an international perspective; its excellence reflects the breadth of their joint knowledge, their sound clinical base, and their familiarity with the literature. I strongly recommend their book to clinicians, teachers, researchers, and students with an interest in that still so-elusive disorder we know as schizophrenia.

Robin M. Murray
May, 2008

Preface

As Professor Murray alludes to in his kind Foreword, this book reflects the knowledge and clinical experience of the authors who have worked on several continents. Accordingly, the book contains information on several medications that may be available in one country but not another. It is important to check medication availability, dosage, and prescribing information with local regulatory and pharmaceutical sources. Additionally, information about medications often changes over time and so readers should consult other sources to verify information or clarify details. Finally, books are only one source of information and can not substitute for the skill and advice of an experienced doctor.

It is our hope that this book will be an aid to people who care for, or live with, people who have this illness. However, it is not intended to be an alternative to the sound advice of a doctor who knows the patients situation. Please bear in mind these considerations as you use this book.

David J. Castle and Peter Buckley

Abbreviations

ACT	Assertive Community Treatment
CDS	Calgary Depression Scale
CATEGO	computerized algorithm
CATIE	Clinical Antipsychotic Trials of Intervention Effectiveness
CB1	cannabinoid CB1
CBT	Cognitive-Behaviour Therapy
CDS	Calgary Depression Scale
COMT	catechol-O-methyl transferase
CT	computerized tomography
CTJ	collaborative treatment journal
CUtLASS	Cost Utility of the Latest Antipsychotic Drugs in Schizophrenia Studies
DSM	US Diagnostic and Statistical Manual of Mental Disorders
DUP	duration of untreated psychosis
ECT	electroconvulsive therapy
EE	expressed emotion
EPSE	extrapyramidal side effect
FEP	first episode psychosis
fMRI	functional Magnetic Resonance Imaging
5-H1AA	5-hydroxyindole acetic acid
H1	histaminergic
ICD	International Classification of Diseases
IgG	immunoglobulin G
IgM	immunoglobulin M
IPSS	International Pilot Study of Schizophrenia
LSD	lysergic acid diethylamide
MRS	magnetic resonance spectroscopy
M1	muscarinic
NAA	N-acetyl-aspartate
NaRIs	Noradrenaline Reuptake Inhibitors
NaSSAs	Noradrenaline and Specific Serotonin Antagonists

NC	neutrophil count
NIDS	neurolept-induced deficit syndrome
NMDA	N-methyl-D-aspartate
NMS	neuroleptic malignant syndrome
OCD	obsessive compulsive disorder
PBCs	pregnancy and birth complications
PCP	phencyclidine
PET	Positron Emission Tomography
PT	personal therapy
RCBF	regional cerebral blood flow
SAD	social anxiety disorder
SAPS	Scales for the Assessment of Positive Symptoms
SANS	Scales for the Assessment of Negative Symptoms
SDS	Schedule for the Deficit Syndrome
SPD	schizotypal personality disorder
SPECT	Single Photon Emission Tomography
SRIs	serotonergic antidepressants
SUD	substance use disorder
TD	Tardive dyskinesia
THC	delta-9-tetrahydrocannabinol
TCAs	tricyclic antidepressants
TMS	transcranial magnetic stimulation
VBR	ventricular brain ratio
WBC	white blood cell
WHO	World Health Organisation

Part 1

The myths and the science

Chapter 1

Diagnosis and classification

> **Key points**
> - The schizophrenia concept has a long and changing history, and our modern constructs still lack external validity.
> - There are no pathognomonic symptoms, signs, or laboratory tests for schizophrenia.
> - There are a number of competing subtypologies of schizophrenia, based either on symptom profiles and/or on putative aetiological parameters.
> - A schizophrenia-like psychosis can onset at pretty much any age, though certain clinical features are more or less common depending on age at onset.

1.1 What is it?

Inevitably, our first question asks what we are actually talking about when we refer to 'schizophrenia'. Thomas Szasz' ironic 'sacred symbol of psychiatry', schizophrenia, remains an enigma, though enhanced understanding of the causes, consequences, and potential treatments are bringing light to the subject. What remains problematic for the field, however, is a lack of agreement about what precisely this putative entity is. Whilst the *US Diagnostic and Statistical Manual of Mental Disorders*, now in its 4th (revised) edition, and the World Health Organization's *International Classification of Diseases* 10th edition (see Table 1.1) have provided a reasonably reliable set of criteria for 'schizophrenia', the validity of the construct remains elusive, and clinicians and researchers need to be wary about accepting these as the definitive constructs. Indeed, schizophrenia remains a clinical diagnosis, based on certain signs and symptoms, and none of these is pathognomonic; there is also no laboratory or radiological test for the disorder as such.

Table 1.1 DSM and ICD diagnoses of schizophrenia	
DSM-IV R	**ICD-10**
Symptoms	*Symptoms*
At least 1 month unless successfullly treated:	At least one of
• Delusions	• Thought echo, insertion, withdrawal, broadcast
• Hallucinations	• Passivity phenomena or delusional perception
• Disorganized speech	• Third person conversing or running commentary hallucinations.
• Disorganized or catatonic behaviour	At least two of
• Negative symptoms	• Persistent hallucinations in any modality, with delusions
At least two symptoms required unless	• Disorganised speech
• Delusions are bizarre	• Catatonia
• Hallucinations (third person conversing or running commentary)	• Negative symptoms (must be 'primary')
Social/Occupational Dysfunction	
• Work	
• Interpersonal relations	
• Self care	
Duration 6 months at least.	*Duration* 1 month at least.
Exclusions	*Exclusions*
• Schizoaffective disorder	• mood disorder
• Bipolar disorder	• organic brain disease
• General medical	• alcohol/drug-related intoxication
• Substance induced	

To see the current conception of schizophrenia in proper context, we need to trace the history of the construct, and understand the ways in which nomenclature, nosology, and definition have changed over time. Box 1.1 provides an overview of early contributions to thinking about schizophrenia, although, as German Berrios has pointed out, there is actually no clear linkage or continuity across these concepts, over time. Furthermore, the meaning of 'dementia' changed over time, such that to Benedict Augustin Morel it did not have any connotation of irreversibility. In any event, it was Emil Kraepelin's contribution to the delineation of what he called 'dementia praecox', which has been most enduring. In fact, his description was of an illness with a male excess, and early onset (usually below the age of 25 years), and an inevitably poor longitudinal course. Kraepelin did not use the label 'dementia' inadvisedly, believing it to be a brain disorder for which the underlying biological basis would eventually be found. His differentiation of dementia praecox from manic depressive psychosis was based largely on contrasting outcomes, with the latter usually showing an episodic course with good inter-morbid functioning.

What is not so well publicized is that Kraepelin understood that these were not the only psychotic illnesses, defining also a later onset paranoid psychosis with a course intermediate between dementia praecox and manic depressive psychosis; he termed this 'paraphrenia', and alluded to other types of psychosis as well. Also, the time of Kraepelin was one where a number of infectious causes of psychotic disorders were highly prevalent, syphilis (the 'great mimicker') being perhaps the most troublesome in clouding and corrupting clinical diagnoses.

It is well known that it was Eugen Bleuler who actually introduced the term 'schizophrenia' (in fact, 'the group of schizophrenias'), from the Greek rather than the Latin route. This term reflected what he considered the key to the understanding of this group of disorders, namely, the 'splitting of the psychic functions'. Bleuler emphasized the importance of symptoms and signs of schizophrenia and delineated them into 'primary' and 'secondary' (see Box 1.2). He saw the former as the core of schizophrenia, with the delusions and hallucinations as 'productive' symptoms.

Box 1.1 The historical antecedents of the schizophrenia concept

- Benedict Augustin Morel (1809–1873): 'demence precoce'
- Karl Kahlbaum (1828–1899): 'catatonia'
- Ewald Hecker (1843–1909): 'hebephrenia'
- Emil Kraepelin (1856–1926): 'dementia praecox' aggregates catatonia, hebephrenia, and 'dementia paranoides'
- Eugen Bleuler (1857–1939): 'the group of schizophrenias'
- Kasanin (1933): 'schizoaffective' disorder
- Kurt Schneider (1887–1967): 'first rank' symptoms
- Karl Leonhard (1960): 'cycloid psychoses'

Box 1.2 Bleuler's primary and secondary symptoms of schizophrenia

Primary (the 'four A's')
- Ambivalence
- Autism
- Disturbance of affect
- Disordered association.

Secondary
- Delusions
- Hallucinations.

In many ways, Bleuler's view of the secondary nature of what are now known as 'positive' psychotic symptoms still makes sense, as we know that delusions and hallucinations can occur in anyone, given certain circumstances, and certainly they, of themselves, carry little or no diagnostic value. For example, a brain tumour, intoxication with cannabis or amphetamines, alcohol withdrawal, temporal lobe epilepsy, and mania and depression can all be associated with hallucinations and delusions. However, there are certain types of positive symptoms that do seem to be more likely to be associated with schizophrenia than with other disorders, and these were grouped by Kurt Schneider and labelled 'first rank' symptoms (Box 1.3). Probably because they could be reliably measured and defined,

---

Box 1.3 Schneider's First Rank Symptoms of schizophrenia

Auditory hallucinatory experiences:

- *Third person auditory hallucinations:* two or more voices discussing the individual in the third person (he, she, it); often derogatory/persecutory
- *Running commentary:* a voice commenting on the person's actual actions, in the third person
- *Audible thoughts* ('gedankenlaudwerten'): hearing one's own thoughts out loud.

Delusional perception:

- A normal percept to which an 'un-understandable' delusional attribution is given; there is usually an immediacy about the attribution, unlike in delusions of reference.

Passivity phenomena:

- A series of phenomena where the person experiences their *will, actions, affect, or bodily (somatic) functions* are 'taken over' by some alien influence; an 'as if' phenomenon, such as: 'It is as though my actions are controlled by a robot; I feel like a puppet on a string.'

Permeability of ego boundaries:

- *Thought insertion:* not all thoughts in one's mind are one's own; thoughts are being 'put into' the person's mind; there may be secondary elaboration, for example, 'An intergalactic machine is putting thoughts into my mind'
- *Thought withdrawal:* the reverse of thought insertion; may be experienced as mind transiently 'going blank'
- *Thought broadcast:* a feeling that thoughts dissipate out of the person's mind and are 'shared' by others; more than just feeling others can 'read my mind.'

Schneider's set of symptoms became widely adopted by the field, though it became increasingly clear that none are actually pathognomonic of schizophrenia, also being seen in patients with mania, for example. Also, they are simply cross-sectional symptoms, and do not encompass any notion of longitudinal course of illness, a feature that defined Kraepelin's dementia praecox.

The issue of longitudinal course and its importance has been re-incorporated into more modern definitions of schizophrenia. However, the duration criterion has been somewhat arbitrarily defined as anything from 2 weeks (in the Research Diagnostic Criteria) to 6 months (in DSM-III and all versions thereafter). Also, the 6 months in DSM can be constructed largely of non-productive symptoms (see Table 1.1), and these can be difficult to differentiate from prodromal or even antecedent developmental or personality problems. The decision as to what constitutes the 'onset' of such symptoms is particularly difficult, as they often emerge from 'normal' functioning in a non-specific way. Also, the imposition of a longitudinal course criterion does land up defining schizophrenia as a certain type of illness, namely one with a relatively poor outcome. It also begs the question of how to label disorders that look like schizophrenia cross-sectionally but do not meet the duration criterion. Again, neatly but arbitrarily, DSM-IV states that such an illness with a duration over a month but less than 6 months should be called 'schizophreniform psychosis'.

1.2 What is it not?

'Organic' psychoses: By definition, schizophrenia as we know it is a disorder of exclusion, in that if a clear 'organic' factor is 'causing' the symptoms and signs, then it is labelled an 'organic' psychosis'. In many ways this is silly, because there is a great deal of evidence (as detailed in the following sections) that schizophrenia is a brain disease and that there are brain abnormalities which can be demonstrated in many individuals with the disorder; there is also a strong suggestion that some of the brain changes are progressive. Also, the exclusion of the so-called drug-induced psychosis does not tally well with the fact that people with a vulnerability to schizophrenia are more prone to the evolution of psychotic symptoms on exposure to certain substances of abuse (see following sections): this suggests 'drug-precipitated' to be a more apposite term in many such cases.

Alcoholic hallucinosis: A syndrome of chronic persecutory hallucinations in clear consciousness, associated with long-term alcohol abuse, creates a particular problem. The label 'alcoholic hallucinosis' is usually applied, but a number of such cases in the longer term evolve into a syndrome that looks indistinguishable from chronic paranoid schizophrenia.

Schizoaffective disorder: Another very contentious issue is the nosological status of so-called schizoaffective disorder. It was Kasanin in the 1930s who described cases of psychosis with schizophrenia-like as well as strong affective features, a direct challenge to the Kraepelinian dichotomy. The field has had considerable difficulty accommodating this group, who have either been effectively denied or defined so narrowly (e.g. DSM-IV-TR: see Table 1.1) such that few cases are so labelled. In clinical practice, however, many individuals are found to have psychotic and affective symptoms, and might indeed change in terms of clinical presentation over time. But such patients tend to be excluded from clinical trials and are overall something of a nosological inconvenience.

Delusional disorder: Another group of 'functional' psychoses that are considered separate from schizophrenia are the delusional disorders. This group is characterized by well-circumscribed delusions in the absence of negative or disorganization symptoms. The delusional content is 'understandable' such as beliefs about having a disease (also termed 'monosymptomatic hypochondriacal delusions') or having an unfaithful partner (delusional jealousy, or 'Othello syndrome').

Axis II disorders: Finally, there is the problem of DSM Axis II ('personality') disorders that really could be considered *formes fruste* of schizophrenia. The most obvious is schizotypal personality disorder, characterized by long-standing eccentricity, social withdrawal, and odd beliefs. This has been shown to occur more commonly in families with schizophrenia itself. The relationship of schizoid personality disorder is less clear, but claims could also be made for it being part of a schizophrenia spectrum.

1.3 Are there subtypes?

Many attempts have been made at subtyping schizophrenia, mostly on the basis of phenomenology and/or longitudinal course. Karl Leonhard, for example, differentiated what he called the 'phasic psychoses' (essentially mood disorders with psychosis) from 'cycloid psychoses', 'unsystematic schizophrenias', and 'systematic schizophrenias'. An overview of this classification system is shown in Box 1.4. It will not surprise the reader that slicing the proverbial pie into so many small pieces was not grasped with alacrity by clinicians or researchers, proving too cumbersome for everyday use. However, clinicians will have come across patients who do seem to 'fit' Leonhard's descriptions: the cycloid psychoses are a case in point.

Box 1.4 Leonhard's classification of 'non-psychic' psychoses

Cycloid psychoses
- Anxiety–happiness psychosis
- Excited–inhibited confusion psychosis
- Hyperkinetic–akinetic motility psychosis.

The unsystematic schizoprenias
- Affect-laden paraphrenia
- Cataphasia (schizophasia)
- Periodic catatonia.

The systematic schizophrenias
Simple systematic schizophrenias
a) catatonic forms
- Parakinetic catatonia
- Affected catatonia
- Proskinetic catatonia
- Negativistic catatonia
- Voluble catatonia
- Sluggish catatonia.

b) hebephrenic forms
- Silly hebephrenia
- Eccentric hebephrenia
- Insipid hebephrenia
- Autistic hebephrenia.

c) paranoid forms
- Hypochondriacal paraphrenia
- Phonemic paraphrenia
- Incoherent paraphrenia
- Fantastic paraphrenia
- Confabulatory paraphrenia
- Expansive paraphrenia.

Combined systematic schizophrenias
- Combined systematic catatonias
- Combined systematic hebephrenias
- Combined systematic paraphrenias.

The current DSM/ICD view is informed (whether directly or indirectly) to some extent by Leonhard's classification, but is much more simple, as shown in Box 1.5. Congruent with the atheoretical approach of DSM, these proposed subtypes are not based on any particular aetiological parameters: indeed, they are essentially judgements of symptom profiles based predominantly on cross-sectional observation. In practice, a typology should at the very least be able to delineate enduring subtypes, but of the DSM subtypes, it is only the 'paranoid' that has reasonable longitudinal stability. Also, 'catatonia' is seen in disorders other than schizophrenia, and it has been argued that it should be considered a type of movement disorder rather than a subtype of schizophrenia (see Box 1.6).

Box 1.5 DSM/ICD subtypes of schizophrenia

- *Paranoid:* delusions and hallucinations but no prominent negative or disorganization symptoms
- *Disorganized (DSM)/Hebephrenic (ICD):* prominent disturbance of affect, volition, and thought stream; ICD states adolescent/young adults only
- *Catatonic:* prominent motoric disturbance (see Box 1.6)
- *Undifferentiated:* meet schizophrenia diagnostic criteria, but not one of the foregoing subtypes
- *Residual:* prominent negative symptoms in the absence of prominent positive symptoms
- *Simple:* slow progression of negative symptoms in the absence of positive symptoms (ICD considers this akin to schizotypal personality disorder).

Box 1.6 Catatonic symptoms

- *Stupor:* clouding of consciousness
- *Excitement:* excessive motor activity
- *Posturing:* odd postures adopted and held for protracted periods
- *Negativism:* performs act 'opposite' to that requested/shown
- *Rigidity:* motor rigidity
- *Waxy flexibility:* 'holds' given posture for protracted periods
- *Automatic obedience:* complies with requests without question
- *Perseveration:* repeated repetition of vocal utterances (echolalia) or motor movements (echopraxia).

We are far away from being able to determine subtypes of schizophrenia on the basis of particular aetiological factors, and in any case multifactorial polygenic models usually pertain with a number of cumulative causal factors acting in synergy with a genetic predisposition (of which more in the following sections). Subtyping on the basis of gender and age at onset has also been proposed, as outlined in Section 1.4.

1.4 Is there a late onset schizophrenia?

Another example of rather arbitrary decision making regarding the definition of schizophrenia is that of age at onset. As outlined in Section 1.3, Kraepelin's cases of dementia praecox tended to have an onset before the mid-20s and certainly before the age of 40 years: the very epithet 'praecox' points to this being an early onset disorder. Age at onset was not specifically stated as a diagnostic criterion until Feighner's criteria were introduced in 1972: they included onset before 40 years as one feature, though technically one could still have onset of illness at any age. It was DSM-III in 1980 that essentially obliterated late-onset schizophrenia, stipulating that onsets after the age of 45 were simply not schizophrenia, and had to be differently labelled. This piece of nonsense was happily abandoned in later versions of DSM, but the thinking still pervades US psychiatry, and late-onset schizophrenia seems only recently to have been resurrected on that side of the Atlantic.

In fact, arguments about age at onset are in any case impacted by the difficulty in accurately determining 'onset', as outlined previously. Also, compelling evidence of abnormalities in motor, verbal, and social functioning in some children who later develop schizophrenia (discussed in detail subsequently) supports the view that schizophrenia (or at least some subtypes of schizophrenia) is consequent upon neurodevelopmental insult. Hence 'onset' is technically at the time of the impact of such insult (which in many cases is genetically mediated, so onset could be considered to be at conception).

The other problem is that what we consider as 'schizophrenia' is almost certainly, as Bleuler recognized, a group of disorders, and it is quite possible that different subtypes (see subsequent text) onset at different ages. For example, reference to age-at-onset curves from samples collected irrespective of onset age (see Figure 1.1) and diagnosed according to different sets of criteria, show a substantial minority 'onsetting' in very late life (i.e. after the age of 60 years). This female-predominant group has particular features (see Box 1.7) and risk factors (see Box 1.8) that suggest they might be a particular sub-group of the schizophrenias.

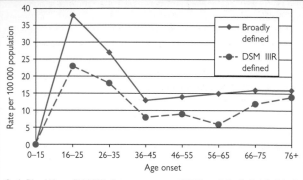

Figure 1.1 Age at onset curves for different definitions of schizophrenia

Castle DJ and Murray RM (1993). *First-contact rates per 100 000 population, for broadly defined & DSM-III-R-defined schizophrenia.* Camberwell, SE London.

Box 1.7 Clinical features of late paraphrenia

Common

- Prominent persecutory delusions
- Organized delusional system common
- Delusional systems dominate daily living
- Partition delusions particularly common (belief that objectively impermeable boundaries such as walls or doors are transgressed to allow access to person's home)
- Hallucinations common and in multiple modalities: visual, auditory (often third person/persecutory/abusive voices), olfactory (e.g. smell of gas being pumped into their home).

Rare

- Negative symptoms almost never occur
- Formal thought disorder extremely uncommon
- Catatonia very rare.

1.5 Does schizophrenia affect males and females similarly?

One of the most consistent findings in the schizophrenia literature is that males tend to have an earlier onset of illness than females. In fact the onset curve for females is not simply pushed to the right in females, and male and female onset curves are not isomorphic. As

Box 1.8 Risk factors for late paraphrenia

- Female gender: major effect (all studies show dramatic female excess)
- Age (by definition: onset usually after 60 years)
- Positive family history of schizophrenia (but less than in early onset)
- Positive family history of affective disorder (some studies only)
- Visual impairment (uncorrected)
- Auditory impairment (uncorrected)
- Premorbid paranoid personality disorder
- Poor premorbid social adjustment
- Reasonable premorbid work adjustment
- Social isolation (considered both casual as well as consequent upon the illness itself).

Figure 1.2 Male and female onset curves for schizophrenia

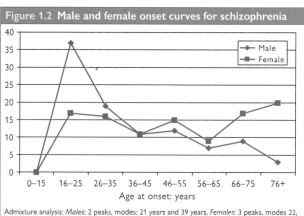

Admixture analysis: *Males*: 2 peaks, modes: 21 years and 39 years, *Females*: 3 peaks, modes 22, 37, and 62 years (Castle *et al.* 1997).

shown in Figure 1.2, males show an early emphatic peak in the late teens to early twenties, followed by a much smaller midlife peak. In females, the early peak is less pronounced, but there is a surge of new cases in midlife and a further peak in very late life.

Much debate has been engaged in, in trying to explain this gender disparity in onset age. This debate needs to be informed by a number of other differences between males and females with schizophrenia. Thus, on aggregate, women with schizophrenia, compared to their male counterparts, are more likely to be married, to have an affective flavour to their illness, to have a lower requirement for antipsychotic medication (at least before the menopause), and to have a more benign longitudinal course of illness, with better symptomatic and psychosocial outcomes.

One way of approaching this is to postulate that some factor delays the onset of schizophrenia and that the better outcomes are consequent upon this. The obvious candidate as a delaying and ameliorating factor is oestrogen, which is known to have antidopaminergic properties and which has been shown in clinical studies to have some impact on acute psychotic symptoms.

Another approach has been to assume that males and females are differentially prone to different subtypes of illness that onset at different ages. For example, it has been suggested that there is a severe early-onset type (similar to Kraepelin's dementia praecox) consequent upon neurodevelopmental insult (all neurodevelopmental disorders are male-predominant); a later onset 'paranoid' type with less negative symptomatology and more affective flavouring, and affecting slightly more females; and a very later onset essentially female disorder with no negative symptoms or formal thought disorder, but florid well-circumscribed delusions and hallucinations in a number of modalities (what has been termed 'late paraphrenia', as outlined earlier).

Chapter 2

Clinical features

2.1 What are the clinical features of schizophrenia?

The current conceptualization of schizophrenia builds on many of the historical themes outlined above. A graphic of the different symptom dimensions is shown in Figure 2.1. A major contribution to this approach to schizophrenia symptomatology was made by Tim Crow in the early 1980s. Crow tried to incorporate two main sets of findings from the then-current research into schizophrenia into a model that essentially linked Bleuler's concept of primary and secondary symptoms, with Kraepelin's view of schizophrenia as a brain disease. Crow took the then-recent findings that people with schizophrenia had a tendency to exhibit, on computerized tomography (CT) scanning, enlarged lateral ventricles and reduced brain grey matter, compared to controls, and suggested that these abnormalities were linked to negative symptoms (similar to Bleuler's four As, but excluding formal thought disorder): he termed this the 'Type 2' symptom dimension. He also postulated that perturbation of dopamine transmission in mesolimbic tracts form the pathogenic basis of positive symptoms (delusions and hallucinations): he labelled these Type 1 symptoms.

The dopamine hypothesis of schizophrenia is presented in more detail in later chapters, as is the evidence for structural brain abnormalities in schizophrenia.

In the United States, Nancy Andreasen took the notion of two symptom sets/dimensions further, and explicitly labelled them 'positive' and 'negative'. She also created a structured assessment interview to elicit the symptoms reliably: the Scales for the Assessment of Positive Symptoms (SAPS) and for Negative Symptoms (SANS): see Boxes 2.1 and 2.2.

Figure 2.1 Symptoms of schizophrenia

Positive	Delusions Hallucinations	Auditory Visual Somatic Olfactory
Negative	Restricted affect Passive social withdrawal Apathy	Primary—part of disease process Secondary to • Depression • Positive symptoms • Antipsychotics
Disorganization	Disorganized actions Formal thought disorder Inappropriate affect	
Cognitive	Executive functioning Verbal fluency Motor speed Working memory	
Depressive	Major depression Demoralization	
Anxiety	Panic Generalized anxiety Social anxiety Obsessive compulsive	

16

Box 2.1 Main domains covered by the Scale for the Assessment of Positive Symptoms (Andreasen 1984)

- Hallucinations
- Delusions
- Bizarre behaviour
- Positive formal thought disorder
- Inappropriate affect.

> **Box 2.2 Main domains covered by the Scale for the Assessment of Positive Symptoms (Andreasen 1984)**
>
> - Affective flattening or blunting
> - Alogia
> - Avolition/apathy
> - Anhedonia-asociality
> - Inattentiveness.

> **Box 2.3 Liddle's model, including underlying functional brain imaging findings (regional cerebral blood flow (RCBF) changes associated with symptom domain)**
>
> Reality distortion (delusions and hallucinations):
> - Increased RCBF: left medial temporal lobe
> - Decreased RCBF: posterior cingulate, left temporoparietal cortex.
>
> Psychomotor poverty (negative symptoms):
> - Increased RCBF: anterior cingulate, thalamus
> - Decreased RCBF: venterolateral prefrontal cortex and insula, and parietal association cortex.
>
> Disorganization (formal thought disorder, inappropriate affect):
> - Increased RCBF: caudate
> - Decreased RCBF: lateral prefrontal cortex and parietal association cortex.

Peter Liddle took this yet further, factor analysing symptom profiles from people with schizophrenia, and exploring the underlying pathophysiology using functional neuroimaging techniques. His model, shown in Box 2.3, has gained substantial currency, and is the way in which most schizophrenia researchers talk about the clinical features of the disorder.

There has been a recent extension of these ideas, whereby it is suggested that the positive symptoms of schizophrenia are consequent upon a hyperdopaminergic state in mesolimbic pathways, and negative symptoms consequent upon a hypodopaminergic state in mesocortical pathways. This notion explains why those older 'typical' antipsychotics which simply block dopamine D2 receptors fairly indiscriminantly are effective for the control of positive symptoms, but make negative symptoms worse. It also provides a model for how partial dopamine D2 receptor antagonists such as aripiprazole can effectively treat positive symptoms by reducing dopamine transmission in the hyperdopaminergic mesolimbic pathways, and also (theoretically at least) ameliorate negative symptoms by enhancing dopamine transmission in hypodopaminergic mesocortical pathways. Of this, more later.

2.2 What about negative symptoms?

Liddle's model is both persuasive and conceptually helpful, but fails adequately to address an important aspect of negative symptoms, namely that they can be consequent upon a number of different causal pathways. It was Will Carpenter and colleagues in the United States who championed the idea of primary and secondary negative symptoms, arguing that the clinical features of negative symptoms can be seen in people who are depressed, people who have received medications that block dopamine D2 receptors (such as the typical antipsychotics), and also in people who are experiencing prominent positive symptoms (see Box 2.4). In their Schedule for the Deficit Syndrome (SDS) Brian Kirkpatrick, Will Carpenter and colleagues stress that 'primary' negative symptoms can be assessed only if secondary causes (as above) are excluded: Box 2.5 outlines the main areas covered by the SDS.

Certainly in clinical practice, secondary negative symptoms are important to be aware of, as they are relatively readily treated (see Box 2.4). Primary negative symptoms are seen prominently in some

Box 2.4 Negative symptoms: treatment strategies

Primary		• Use atypical antipsychotic; • Consider adjunctive treatments (see Chapter 8); • If persistent, consider clozapine.
Secondary	To depression	Antidepressant medication (SSRI or mirtazepine preferred: see Chapter 3) and psychological therapy.
	To positive symptoms	Optimize treatment of positive symptoms: pharmacological and psychosocial approaches should be explored.
	To D2 receptor blockade	• Consider atypical antipsychotic; • If persistent EPSE on atypical antipsychotic, consider adjunctive anticholinergic agent.

Box 2.5 Main domains covered by the Schedule for the Deficit Syndrome (SDS) (Kirkpatrick et al. 1989)

- Affective flattening or blunting
- Alogia
- Avolition-apathy
- Anhedonia-asociality
- Attention.

patients (notably those with the so-called deficit syndrome), and tend to be much more difficult to treat (clozapine and low-dose amisulpride might have a particular place here, as detailed in Part 2 of this book). Also, it is negative symptomatology that tends to drive disability in schizophrenia, in social and vocational spheres.

2.3 What about cognitive functioning?

Considerable importance has been placed on the cognitive deficits that occur in some people with schizophrenia. In many ways these deficits, along with negative symptoms, are the 'last frontier' in the treatment of schizophrenia, as the antipsychotic medications we have show but modest and inconsistent effects on cognitive functioning. Also it seems clear that cognitive deficits result in a significant amount of the disability associated with the illness, notably in terms of work and study.

Kraepelin's label of 'dementia' implies a progressive decline in cognitive functioning, but there is debate as to how much of the cognitive deficit in schizophrenia is progressive, and how much of it is a relatively static accompaniment of the predisposition to the illness. Thus, it is well established that people who later develop schizophrenia (especially severe early onset schizophrenia, and expressly in males) show deficits in IQ that antedate the manifestation of positive symptoms. Indeed, birth cohort studies have shown non-specific deficits in motor, verbal, and social domains even very early in life, in those destined to later develop schizophrenia. Of course these findings are very non-specific, and there are many people with schizophrenia who do not show such antecedent problems, but at an aggregate level the findings suggest that impeded cognitive functioning is a core part of the illness, and is present way before the onset of positive psychotic symptoms.

Having said this, there is also evidence that, in some people at least, cognitive functioning continues to deteriorate as the illness progresses: this has been most dramatically shown in elderly schizophrenia patients by Phil Harvey and colleagues. There is much conjecture about the explanation for this finding, but a number of general factors should be considered, including 'institutionalization' (which occurs even in these days of community care, with many people with schizophrenia experiencing social isolation and having a sparse network with whom to engage in cognitive tasks such as conversation), nutritional problems, physical health problems, and exposure to alcohol and illicit drugs. Also, some of the older antipsychotics actually seem to have the propensity to make cognitive dysfunction worse, and other prescribed agents such as anticholinergics and benzodiazepines can also have detrimental effects on cognitive functioning.

> ## Box 2.6 Domains of cognitive functioning impaired in schizophrenia (adapted from Wykes and Castle 2008)
>
> Mild impairment
> - Perceptual skills
> - Delayed recognition memory
> - Verbal and full-scale IQ.
>
> Moderate impairment
> - Distractibility
> - Memory and working memory
> - Delayed recall.
>
> Severe impairment
> - Executive functioning
> - Verbal fluency
> - Motor speed.

Not all domains of cognitive functioning are impaired to the same extent in people with schizophrenia, as shown in Box 2.6. Individual assessment is required to profile the neurocognitive difficulties of each patient, in order to understand the impact of such deficits on their daily life and to inform treatment interventions: treatments are discussed in more detail in Part 2 of this book.

2.4 Are people with schizophrenia violent?

One of the very unfortunate consequences of deinstitutionalization has been that many more people with schizophrenia have fallen foul of the criminal justice system and languish in prison, where they are vastly over-represented. Also, a few cases of homicide perpetrated by people with schizophrenia have received notoriety and extensive publicity, serving to increase stigma amongst the general population, and to further marginalize people with a severe mental illness.

The truth is that any increase in violent crime associated with schizophrenia in the era after deinstitutionalization has been mirrored by an overall increase in such crimes amongst the general population. Also, the vast majority of people with schizophrenia are neither violent nor given to criminality. And the associations of violent crime in people with schizophrenia are much the same as those associated with violent crime in the general population, as shown in Box 2.7. The exception is those particular phenomena that occur in some individuals with schizophrenia and which might be directly related to violent acts. Perhaps the most well recognized are delusional jealousy and 'command' hallucinations, where the individual hears a voice or voices telling him to perpetrate a certain act.

Box 2.7 **Associations of violence in people with schziophrenia**

General
- Previous violence
- Previous forensic history
- Sociopathy
- Male gender
- Adolescence/young adulthood
- Alcohol and/or illicit substance use.

Symptom-related
- Paranoid delusions
- Delusional jealousy
- Command hallucinations.

Some clinician researchers have suggested that it is not so much any one symptom that should raise concern, but rather when certain symptoms come together: the so-called 'threat-control-override' symptom complex. This collection of symptoms includes command hallucinations, persecutory delusions, and experiences of external control. Obviously all such features—both as individual symptoms and as symptom profiles—should be screened for along with the other general risk factors in any risk assessment exercise. It is also true that the risk of violence is typically increased when somebody is floridly ill and the risk is low in patients whose symptoms are well controlled. This underlines the importance of optimal control of psychotic symptoms in a consistent and ongoing way, with regular clinical monitoring.

Chapter 3

Comorbidity

Key points

- Comorbid symptoms are common in people with schizophrenia, but are often missed by clinicians and not adequately treated.
- Depressive comorbidity might be dismissed as negative symptomatology unless specific features are enquired about.
- Depression is associated with suicidality.
- Anxiety disorders comorbid with schizophrenia are generally associated with poorer longitudinal course for both disorders.
- Obsessive compulsive disorder can be precipitated or worsened by most of the atypical antipsychotics.
- The use of alcohol and illicit substances is common in people with schizophrenia, and results in more relapses and hospitalizations, and numerous psychosocial problems.
- The medical health of people with schizophrenia is often poor, and cardiovascular risk factors, in particular, add to the risk of early death.

3.1 What are 'comorbid' symptoms?

Comorbidity is generally taken to refer to the co-occurrence of more than one disorder in the same individual. Our hierarchical approach to psychiatric nosology is such that we tend to see schizophrenia as a disorder that 'trumps' others, and it is always important to be aware of the likelihood of other disorders occurring in someone with schizophrenia. This is more than a semantic problem, as in truth affective and anxiety symptoms are often part and parcel of the clinical presentation and certainly cause distress to the individual and carry disability. In an hierarchical approach where positive and negative symptoms are given primacy, such comorbid symptoms can be dismissed as merely part of the manifestation of 'schizophrenia'. A good example is the tacit assumption that a lack of socialization in people with schizophrenia is due to negative symptomatology, whilst many such individuals actually have social anxiety disorder that can effectively be treated in its own right.

Depression is certainly common in people with schizophrenia, and can be difficult to disentangle from core features of schizophrenia. Depressive symptoms are thought to occur in over 70% of people with schizophrenia, and around one in four would meet criteria for major depressive disorder at some time in their life. Recognition and treatment are critical, as depression is treatable, and if untreated can lead to an extra burden for the individual, and is associated with suicide (which itself is much more common in schizophrenia than the general population: see p. 25). Depression also needs to be differentiated from demoralization, although they can also occur together. Some clinical pointers to making a diagnosis of depression in schizophrenia are given in Box 3.1. It is also worth considering using the Calgary Depression Scale (CDS) of Don Addington and co-workers (Box 3.2), as it was devised specifically for use in people with schizophrenia.

Box 3.1 Diagnostic pointer to depression in schizophrenia

- Vegetative symptoms (anorexia, insomnia)
- Functional shift symptoms (early morning wakening, mood worse in the mornings)
- Low self-esteem
- Guilt
- Suicidality.

Box 3.2 Domains covered by the Calgary Depression Scale for Schizophrenia (CDS) (Addington et al. 1990)

Subjective (based on patient response to set questions):
- Depressed mood
- Hopelessness
- Self-deprecation
- Guilty ideas of reference
- Pathological guilt
- Morning depression
- Early wakening
- Suicidality.

Objective (based on observer observations during the interview):
- Observed depression.

Up to 1 in 20 people with schizophrenia end their lives by suicide. Unlike in other conditions such as alcoholism, where suicide typically occurs after many years when the person has hit 'rock bottom', the typical situation for suicide in schizophrenia is a young man who has been recently diagnosed and has become depressed by the way schizophrenia has changed his life. Depression is the strongest risk factor for suicide in people with schizophrenia and so it is very important to enquire about depressive symptoms (and not to 'misattribute' them to negative symptoms) when patients are clinically assessed: the routine use of self-report mood rating scales can be particularly helpful in terms of longitudinal tracking of symptoms. Also, clearly when a patient hears voices telling him to kill himself or do bizarre dangerous things (e.g. to jump out of a moving car) these symptoms also place the person at higher risk of violent death (either intentional or unintentional).

Of the *anxiety disorders*, panic disorder, generalized anxiety disorder, agoraphobia, and social phobia have all been shown to occur in excess in association with schizophrenia (see Box 3.3). They can all add to distress and disability, and should be recognized and treated appropriately. Happily, psychological and pharmacological treatments proved effective for these disorders not occurring comorbidly are often effective in the context of schizophrenia, though psychological techniques might need to be adapted somewhat and care should be taken in the use of certain antidepressants, as they may interact with antipsychotic agents.

Post-traumatic stress disorder is also more common in people with schizophrenia. In part, this reflects the fact that many such individuals have led disadvantaged and difficult lives, with child sexual abuse having an acknowledged association with adult schizophrenia. The other consideration is that the symptoms of psychosis themselves, along with the trauma all too often associated with the treatment process (notably restraint and seclusion in acute hospital settings) can also be associated with post-traumatic symptoms. In this latter

Box 3.3 Best estimate rates of anxiety disorders in schizophrenia (adapted from Pokos and Castle 2006)	
Generalized anxiety disorder	10–20%
Panic disorder	5–20%
Agoraphobia	5–20%
Social anxiety disorder	25–30%
Specific phobia	5–15%
Obsessive-compulsive disorder	10–15% early psychosis
	20–30% chronic schizophrenia
Any anxiety disorder	**± 50%**

context, prevention is the best strategy, and programmes to reduce the use of restraint and seclusion are welcome: at the very least, the patient should be afforded the opportunity to ventilate their feelings about any such intervention, and be empowered to be included in planning how better to manage such clinical scenarios should they arise in the future.

Obsessive compulsive disorder (OCD) has an interesting association with schizophrenia. Many studies have reported that it is common in people with schizophrenia, but there has been some debate as to causal pathways and implications for longitudinal course and for treatment. Thus, Stengel argued that such symptoms could help to 'make sense' and control the symptoms of psychotic breakdown, but subsequent work has tended to show the obverse, namely that OC symptoms are associated with a poor longitudinal trajectory in schizophrenia: indeed, some authors have suggested that there is a particularly pernicious 'schizo-obsessive disorder'. Another twist is that the atypical antipsychotics that antagonize serotonin 5-HT2 receptors have been associated with exacerbations and/or de-novo evolution of OC symptoms in some people. Again, these are all too often missed clinically, as they are thought to reflect psychotic processes. In reality, they can be effectively treated using psychological and pharmacological paradigms (serotonergic antidepressants (SSRIs)), with the caveats about drug–drug interactions outlined above. Ironically, atypical antipsychotics have an established place, as adjuncts to SSRIs (and sometimes as sole agents), in the treatment of OCD itself.

26

3.2 Why is substance abuse comorbidity so damaging?

It is widely accepted that there is a significant overlap between the use of alcohol and illicit substances, and schizophrenia. Worldwide, rates of substance use disorder (SUD) in people with schizophrenia aggregate around 40–60%, with higher rates reported in many clinical sites. Alcohol is the most widely used substance, followed by cannabis. Rates of other substance use largely follow general population rates, with amphetamines being common in countries like Australia, and cocaine in the United States.

It can be difficult for clinicians to differentiate between drug-induced and 'primary' psychotic disorders. Box 3.4 provides some guidelines, but it should be borne in mind that there is often a mix of factors, including underlying biological vulnerability that makes some people more vulnerable to the psychomimetic actions of illicit substances: as stated previously, the term substance-precipitated psychosis might be a more accurate term in this situation.

> **Box 3.4 Factors suggesting a primary rather than substance-induced psychosis (based on Lubman and Sundram 2003)**
>
> - Psychotic symptoms antedate the substance use.
> - Withdrawal of the substance of abuse does not halt psychotic symptoms (may need up to a month for substances such as cannabis to 'wash out').
> - Psychotic symptoms continue during times of prolonged abstinence.
> - The types of psychotic symptoms are not those usually seen in association with the particular substance used.
> - There is a family history of a primary psychotic illness.

The reasons why people with schizophrenia use illicit substances include the following:

- Alleviation of 'negative affect', such as dysphoria, boredom, and anxiety
- Social affiliation (to be with others, to fit in) and
- Enhancement (to get high, to have fun).

These factors are no different from those that drive substance use in people without a mental illness; it is just that those with schizophrenia have higher rates of all of these risk factors. Of interest is that 'self-medication' of positive symptoms and side effects of medication are not major reasons for SUD in schizophrenia: if the self-medication hypothesis holds true, it pertains to negative and affective rather than positive psychotic symptoms.

Irrespective of reasons for use, the problematic use of alcohol and illicit substances has profound negative implications for the longitudinal course of schizophrenia. This has been shown in many studies, and is obvious to clinicians. The extent of damage that SUD can do in schizophrenia is detailed in Box 3.5.

A better understanding of SUD in schizophrenia, and in particular more effective treatments, is a major priority to mental health and drug and alcohol clinicians and policy-makers. The existing and developing treatments are detailed in Part 2 of this book.

3.3 What about physical comorbidity?

As already stated, suicide is a major risk in schizophrenia, and far too many people with the disorder die by their own hand. Death by other violent means is also more common for this group. But these tragic outcomes are not the major contributors to the fact that people with schizophrenia die on average 10–20 years younger than their non-mentally ill counterparts.

Box 3.5 Impact of problematic substance use on outcomes in schizophrenia

Mental health issues
- Increased psychotic symptoms
- Greater relapse rates
- Higher hospitalization rates
- Frequent emergency contacts with mental health services
- Reduced adherence to treatment
- Higher attempted and completed suicide rates.

Violence and crime
- Increased violence
- Elevated crime rates
- Increased rates of incarceration.

Physical health
- Poorer overall health care and nutrition
- Increased specific physical health risks including HIV, hepatitis C
- Overall increased mortality.

Finances and vocation
- Financial problems directly and indirectly related to drug use
- Instability of work/studies.

Housing and families
- Unstable accommodation
- Homelessness
- Increased family conflict.

A wide range of physical health problems occur in excess in people with schizophrenia. Regrettably, these dangerous and potentially life-shortening illnesses are all too often neither adequately recognized nor optimally treated. Added to this is the knowledge that many of the medications prescribed for mental health problems have side effects that exacerbate cardiovascular risk factors, as detailed in the following section.

Cardiovascular risk factors: Cardiovascular deaths are the major single cause of death in people with schizophrenia. Factors contributing to risk include those shown in Box 3.6. These are all seen in excess amongst people with schizophrenia, and contribute to overall cardiovascular risk in an additive manner.

Obesity: Weight gain is a major issue for people with schizophrenia, mediated, *inter alia*, by a sedentary lifestyle; a diet dominated by high carbohydrate foods; alcohol abuse; and the effect of prescribed medications. The antipsychotics clozapine and olanzapine have been

> **Box 3.6 Cardiovascular risk factors (adapted from Meyer 2003)**
>
> - Elevated total cholesterol
> - Hypertension
> - Cigarette smoking
> - Being overweight/obese
> - Sedentary lifestyle/lack of exercise
> - Diabetes.

particularly implicated, but quetiapine and risperidone can also cause a degree of weight gain (see Chapter 8); aripiprazole and ziprasidone appear mostly to be 'weight neutral'. Other medications such as sodium valproate and lithium, which are often used adjunctively in people with schizophrenia, are also associated with weight gain and can add to the burden. Weight gain adds to cardiovascular risk, as detailed earlier, but also impacts people's body image and self-esteem, and adds to the stigma of having a mental illness.

Diabetes: Rates of type 2 diabetes are rising globally, and people with schizophrenia are at particular risk. An elevated risk of diabetes in people with schizophrenia has been described for decades, and antedates the discovery of antipsychotic medications. However, it is clear that some antipsychotics are associated with particularly heightened rates of diabetes. Of the typical agents, the phenothiazines are particularly implicated; of the atypical agents, clozapine and olanzapine carry the highest risk. For example, in a 5-year study of 101 patients on clozapine, there were 36 new cases of diabetes and people with existing diabetes showed an exacerbation of their condition. The precise mechanisms are complex, with central adiposity being a contributing factor, but a direct diabetogenic effect also operating. Thus, care should be taken in the use of agents known to increase the risk of diabetes, particularly in those with other risk factors for diabetes (see Box 3.7). Monitoring guidelines and a proforma are provided in the following sections.

Hyperlipidaemia: Elevated levels of total cholesterol and triglycerides, and low levels of high-density lipoprotein are associated with increased risk of cardiovascular disease. People with schizophrenia are prone to abnormalities of serum lipids because of factors including poor diet and a sedentary lifestyle, but certain antipsychotics, notably the phenothiazines and dibenzodiazepines, are particularly implicated. Again, monitoring is important, as is dietary advice and, if these are ineffective, switching to another antipsychotic and/or the use of a lipid-lowering agent should be considered.

Cancer: Cancer mortality rates overall are higher in people with schizophrenia, compared to the general population. Lifestyle and

Box 3.7 Risk factors for Type 2 diabetes
General
• Genetic predisposition
• Abdominal obesity
• Excess caloric intake
• Diet high in fats
• Low physical activity.
Antipsychotic-related
• Increased appetite, especially for 'junk' food
• Altered fat distribution (abdominal obesity)
• Decreased physical activity due to sedation
• Direct effects on insulin cascade, free fatty acids.

health-seeking behaviours probably play a major role here. There is some debate about the risk of specific cancers, but breast and gastrointestinal malignancies are fairly consistently found to be elevated. Lung cancer rates are probably not as high as one might expect in a group who has such high rates of cigarette smoking, and a putative 'protective' effect of antipsychotics and/or the illness itself have been posited, though lack confirmation: it might simply be that they die earlier of other causes such as cardiovascular disease. What is undoubtedly the case is that people with schizophrenia are less likely to have regular screening for cancers, and tend not to receive optimal treatments.

Chapter 4

Epidemiology and longitudinal course

Key points

- Schizophrenia afflicts all known human societies at roughly the same rate at a broad population level, though there is significant variation within populations.
- The outcome for the disorder is variable, but a significant minority of patients have a poor symptomatic and psychosocial outcome.
- Ameliorable factors associated with a poor outcome in schizophrenia include lack of medication adherence, illicit substance use, and high family conflict.
- Obtaining paid permanent employment is a major problem for people with schizophrenia, due to illness factors as well as workplace and societal factors.

4.1 How common is schizophrenia?

The answer to this question is bedevilled by changes in diagnostic practice over time, between sites and across studies. Indeed, at one time there was so little consistency in the definition that rates of schizophrenia in the United States were notably much higher than in the United Kingdom. The quip was that one could elicit a cure for schizophrenia in a New Yorker by putting them on a flight to Heathrow. The inherent nonsense of this situation was shown scientifically in the landmark US–UK diagnostic project, which compared rates of schizophrenia in London and New York using an agreed set of criteria, determined on the basis of a computerised algorithm (CATEGO) driven by symptom sets defined using a standardized questionnaire, the Present State Examination (PSE: then in its 9th revision). The fact that this rigorous approach showed that Londoners were in fact just as likely as New Yorkers to meet criteria for schizophrenia led to a major revision of thinking in US psychiatry, and was instrumental in the evolution of operationalized criteria for schizophrenia. These criteria have changed in emphasis and stringency over time, as outlined earlier. The most recent evolutions are DSM-IV (text revision) and ICD-10 (see Box 1.1).

So, if the United States and United Kingdom have very similar rates of schizophrenia, what about rates in other parts of the world? The Word Health Organisation (WHO) undertook to study this, and set up an incidence and prevalence study (the International Pilot Study of Schizophrenia, or IPSS) across nine countries, using the PSE. Because of vastly different health service structures across the different settings, the sampling frame was inclusive of a wide variety of agencies (e.g. non-government organizations) and individuals (e.g. indigenous healers) who might be accessed by people with schizophrenia. The results of the study were remarkable in that (1) the rate of stringently defined schizophrenia showed only a twofold variation across sites (from 7–14 per 100 000 per year); and (2) the outcome appeared to be better for those in developing countries. This latter finding was largely confirmed by the subsequent WHO 'Ten Country Study'.

Prevalence studies (i.e. reporting the number of cases in a given population at a given point in time—point prevalence; or over a set period—period prevalence) have also been remarkably similar in their outcomes, when they have used appropriate methods, including operational criteria for diagnosis. Thus, modern general population studies from the United States, the United Kingdom, and Australia have all reported rates of around 0.5–1.5%; the lower figure is more consistent with the total international literature. Another way of expressing these figures is that of 'lifetime morbid risk', that is, the risk at birth of anyone developing the illness, all else being equal; this is usually rounded to 0.5–1.0%.

In fact schizophrenia is not entirely uniform in its distribution. Although we know of no society where the illness is never seen, there is considerable variation in prevalence rates; for example, high rates have been found in Northern Sweden and possibly Western Ireland, and in deprived inner-city areas in large cities. The latter finding was first conclusively shown by Faris and Dunham in 1920s Chicago, where high prevalence areas in the deprived inner city were circled by concentrically lower prevalence areas reflecting suburbs with high socio-economic status. Such patterns have been nicely mapped in modern times in Nottingham, UK. The question is whether people with schizophrenia simply 'drift' down the social scale into such areas as a consequence of the illness itself, or whether there is something pernicious about deprived inner city areas that is associated with increased risk of schizophrenia. Probably both effects operate, and Preben Mortensen and colleagues have shown convincingly that being brought up in a large city in Denmark was associated with a heightened risk of later schizophrenia, compared to a small-town or rural upbringing.

What is also very clear is that migrants are at greater risk of schizophrenia. This has been strikingly and consistently demonstrated in the African-Caribbean population in the United Kingdom, where the first and second generations both show higher rates (up to 10-fold and 14-fold, respectively) than either native-born Whites or African-Caribbeans who stayed in the Caribbean. Similarly, high rates have been shown in Surinamese migrants to The Netherlands. The precise reasons for this effect are not clear, with biological (e.g. exposure to novel viruses) and psychosocial (e.g. migration stress and the experience of discrimination in the adopted country) influences being cited. The importance of psychosocial parameters is underlined by findings that those at highest risk of schizophrenia are Blacks moving into predominantly White neighbourhoods in predominantly White countries.

4.2 Is it getting rarer?

There is ongoing debate about whether schizophrenia has been a universal accompaniment of the human condition, or is a disease that came into being in the late eighteenth century. The latter view has been promulgated by, amongst others, Edward Hare, and is known as the 'recency hypothesis'. The idea is that some sort of biological change occurred to humans at that time, resulting in the disease. Counter to that, Tim Crow has advocated that schizophrenia is 'the price humans pay for language' and is a by-product of an early 'speciation event' in human evolution. In many ways these arguments are esoteric and impossible to prove one way or another.

More recent trends in the disease are, however, amenable to scientific investigation, albeit with the methodological limitations arising from, *inter alia*:

- Diagnostic habits having changed over time (see Section 4.1 and Chapter 1)
- Sampling frames having been inconsistent (e.g. some studies have used only hospitalized patients, whilst others have relied on case registers), and
- Changes having occurred in service provision (e.g. de-institutionalization).

Despite these caveats, a number of studies have elegantly shown that rates of schizophrenia have declined somewhat over the last 30 years, in a number of developed countries. This finding has not been universal, however, and some investigators have reported static or even increasing rates. In South East London, for example, rates ascertained through a case register, and controlling for changes in the general population over time, actually rose over the 20 years after the mid-1960s; this effect was largely accounted for by an influx into the area of African-Caribbeans, who, as outlined earlier, showed a greater vulnerability to the illness than the indigenous White population.

4.3 Is the long-term outcome inevitably poor?

Initial descriptions of schizophrenia implied a poor longitudinal trajectory, but follow-up studies have now shown the extent of heterogeneity in outcome associated with this diagnostic label. From such studies we can glean that around a quarter of cases have a single episode and return to good psychosocial functioning; around a third have an episodic course with reasonably good inter-morbid functioning; and 40% tend to have a poor outcome.

Certain factors do tend to be associated with a poor outcome in schizophrenia. Some of these are potentially remediable, others are not (see Box 4.1). Clearly services should be configured to deliver optimal care over the lifetime of the illness, and remediable predictors of poor outcome should be targeted expressly. Medication adherence is perhaps the most important single such issue, and this topic is covered in Part 2 of this book. Addressing substance use comorbidity is also vital, as there is a strong association with poor outcomes across a range of domains (see Box 3.5), and there is some evidence (not universal) that stopping illicit substances results in a better outcome than in those who never used in the first place (perhaps a reflection of poor pre-morbid social functioning in this latter group).

Two social factors are worthy of particular mention, namely family environment and life events. *Family environment* came under particular scrutiny during the 1970s, with the observation that certain aspects of family interaction are associated with worse outcome in people with schizophrenia. These factors have been labelled 'expressed emotion' or 'EE', and comprise the elements shown in Box 4.2. Families should, of course, not be blamed as causing poor outcomes for their family member, but can be usefully engaged to change aspects of family dynamics that contribute to the high EE environment. Such work, pioneered by Julian Leff and colleagues in the UK and Gerry Hogarty and colleagues in the United States, has been shown to be effective across a number of cultures, and to be capable of reducing relapse rates in the affected individual.

Life events, on the other hand, are events that occur during the course of a person's life and which might impact on risk of relapse. Usually a distinction is made between life events that occur as a result of becoming ill (e.g. losing a job because of increasing paranoia and inability to concentrate on tasks) and those that are causally associated with relapse (e.g. death of a loved one). The importance of mapping life events and understanding their impact on schizophrenia relapse lie in the ability to help the individual plan for and deal more effectively with such events should they occur. This is linked

Box 4.1 Factors associated with a poor outcome in schizophrenia

Factors not subject to amelioration

- Male gender
- Early onset of illness
- Strong family loading for schizophrenia
- Insidious onset of illness
- Long prodrome
- Poor pre-morbid functioning
- Lack of affective symptoms at onset
- Prominent negative symptoms at onset
- Lack of obvious precipitating factors at onset
- Neurological soft signs
- Significant neurocognitive deficits at onset
- Structural brain abnormalities (somewhat inconsistent findings).

Factors potentially addressed by optimal clinical care

- Long duration of untreated psychosis (debated)
- Suboptimal treatment of psychotic symptoms
- Suboptimal treatment of comorbid symptoms
- Poor medication adherence
- Medication side effects (e.g. neuroleptic-induced deficit syndrome)
- Substance abuse
- High family expressed emotion.

Box 4.2 Elements of family expressed emotion (EE)

- Expressed hostility
- High number of critical comments
- Over-involvement.

with heightening awareness of early warning signs of relapse and intervention strategies to help avoid a full-blown relapse. Strategies to do this are provided in Part 2 of this book.

4.4 How should we define 'remission'?

Definitions of remission in schizophrenia have been inconsistent and usually reflect the clinician's perspective. A useful attempt at standardizing a definition of remission has been provided by Nancy Andreasen and colleagues (see Box 4.3). If this approach is validated and taken up universally, it will allow a much better comparison across studies, and assist in determining the most effective long-term interventions for schizophrenia.

Box 4.3 **Proposed consensus criteria for remission in schizophrenia (from Andreasen et al. 2005)**

A score of mild or less simultaneously on all the following items, for at least 6 months:

Psychoticism (reality distortion)
- Delusions
- Hallucinations.

Disorganization
- Disorganized speech
- Grossly disorganized, bizarre or catatonic behaviour.

Negative symptoms (psychomotor poverty)
- Negative symptoms (encompassing: flat/blunted affect, apathy/asociality/social withdrawal, alogia/lack of spontaneity).

Box 4.4 **Barriers for people with schizophrenia obtaining work**
- Limited access to vocational or educational training
- The debilitating effects of psychiatric symptoms
- Cognitive impairments associated with the illness
- Side effects of medications (e.g. sedation)
- Job design problems
- Lack of support in work environments
- Stigma associated with schizophrenia.

4.5 What prevents people with schizophrenia obtaining work?

Work has great potential benefits for people in general, and is arguably expressly important for people with schizophrenia, as they are often marginalized and dislocated from society. Indeed, it has been shown that people with a mental illness who work have greater self-esteem, better overall life satisfaction, and feel more financially secure. It is thus a travesty that so few people with schizophrenia are in full-time employment.

Reasons for exclusion of people with schizophrenia from the workforce is a consequence of a number of factors including some inherent in the illness itself, some related to the potential workplace, and some a reflection of reduced expectations regarding work capability. Identified barriers are shown in Box 4.4. Suggestions for negotiating these barriers are provided in Part 2 of this book.

Chapter 5

Aetiology

5.1 What causes schizophrenia?

Conventionally the approach to this question is that there are genetic and environmental factors implicated in the causation of schizophrenia. It is increasingly obvious, however, that these are not discrete, and that genes impact environment and vice versa. There are glimpses of how this might operate at an individual level, for example, through knowledge that people with certain genetic variants of the *catechol-O-methyl transferase* (*COMT*) gene (involved in the breakdown of dopamine) are more vulnerable to the manifestation of a schizophreniform psychosis if they consume cannabis. In the case of cannabis abuse, it may well be that people may abuse drugs because of fundamental impairments in the ability to experience pleasure that are due to dysregulation of dopamine, especially in the 'pleasure-seeking'/'sensation craving' region of the brain—the nucleus accumbens. There is growing evidence for dopamine deficiency and/or dysregulation of dopamine as a mechanism underlying addictions. This may also be relevant to how people (who are vulnerable) become psychotic apparently due to cannabis (see Section 5.3). It is also important to appreciate that whatever factors are at work, the mixture of these may be different for each patient. Some researchers then consider schizophrenia as a 'final common pathway' that may occur through a variety of 'insults', acting either alone or together (in various combinations perhaps).

Having said all this, we cannot but commence this section by providing an overview of the genetic contribution to causality, as it is by far the most powerful of the known causal factors. Thus, as Gottesman and Shields usefully summarized, there is a gradient of risk according to the proximity of the genetic relationship to the proband with schizophrenia (see Box 5.1). The closest genetic relationship is to a monozygotic twin, but the 50% discordance in these genetically 'identical' individuals is universally cited as evidence for 'environmental' causal factors. As articulated above, this dichotomous thinking is simplistic, but it is a useful enough starting point to measure what precisely is inherited and what is not, in terms of factors predisposing to schizophrenia. An example is the elegant neuroimaging study by Sudath and colleagues, of monozygotic twins discordant for schizophrenia, which showed greater ventricle-to-brain ratios in the affected compared to the non-affected of each twin pair.

Another interesting twist to the monozygotic twin story is that the offspring of the unaffected twin still carry an elevated risk of schizophrenia. Thus, what is inherited is a degree of vulnerability which then interacts with other factors to result in the manifestation of the illness in some individuals. We also know that some of the vulnerability might show itself as a *forme fruste*; that is, people exhibit some features of schizophrenia but do not meet diagnostic criteria for the illness itself. The most obvious in such a group are those with

---

Box 5.1 Gradient of genetic risk for schizophrenia

- General population risk: ~1%
- Uncle, aunt, nephew or niece with schizophrenia: ~3%
- Grandparent with schizophrenia: ~4%
- Brother or sister with schizophrenia: ~10%
- Dizygotic twin with schizophrenia: ~10%
- One parent with schizophrenia: ~13%
- Both parents with schizophrenia: ~46%
- Monozygotic twin with schizophrenia: ~50%

schizotypal personality disorder (SPD), characterized by social awk-wardness and withdrawal, and odd thinking. SPD is seen in excess amongst the relatives of people with schizophrenia, and people with SPD show abnormalities of cognitive functioning and impaired P-300 latencies on evoked potential testing: these abnormalities are similar to those seen in schizophrenia, but less severe. Furthermore, it seems that some other family members of people with schizophrenia do not exhibit any clinical features of the illness at all, but do show subtle deviations from the norm on specific testing of brain function, including saccadic eye movements and P-300 evoked potentials.

With the molecular genetic revolution, attempts have been made to find the 'schizophrenia gene'. It should be obvious from the foregoing that such a quest is futile, as the condition itself is hetero-geneous, and inheritance is non-Mendelian, with gene–environment interactions and epigenetic effects to boot. This does not mean that the molecular genetic study of schizophrenia has been useless, but it does mean that we need to be looking for genes that act in concert with other genes as well as various environmental factors, to pro-duce the schizophrenia phenotype. One set of genes that have been subject to particular scrutiny are those that govern neurodevelop-ment. These include dysbindin (chromosome 6p22.3), neuregulin (chromosome 8p21–22), and disrupted in schizophrenia 1 (DISC1; chromosome 1q42). The *COMT* gene has also attracted interest, as outlined earlier.

5.2 What 'non-genetic' factors contribute to the risk for schizophrenia?

Factors that have been posited as increasing the risk of schizophrenia are summarized in Box 5.2. Most of these factors have been impli-cated on the basis of epidemiological studies, often aggregated at the population level and thus prone to various methodological prob-lems including the ecological fallacy and residual confounding. Also, association does not of course necessarily betoken causality, and it is as well to remind oneself of the criteria that the British epidemiolo-gist Sir Bradford Hill suggested should be considered in cases of supposed causality (Box 5.3).

Seasonality of birth: An excess of schizophrenia in individuals born in later winter/early spring has been reported form a number of Northern hemisphere countries, but such an effect has not been convincingly shown for the Southern hemisphere. A number of po-tential methodological criticisms have been levelled at the Northern hemisphere findings, including that an age-cohort effect might be operating, such that people born in the at-risk months have more

Box 5.3 Summary of putative 'non-genetic' casual factors in schizophrenia

- Season of birth (late winter, early spring): Northern hemisphere only
- Exposure to influenza type A2 during second trimester of gestation
- Maternal starvation during first trimester of pregnancy
- Pregnancy and birth complications
- Maternal stress during pregnancy
- Urban birth/upbringing
- Migration
- Ethnic minorities
- Substance abuse
- Advancing paternal age.

Box 5.4 Bradford-Hill's causality pointers

- Strength of association (i.e. high odds ratio/risk ratio)
- Consistency of association, across sites and populations
- Specificity of association:
  - specificity of cause
  - specificity of effect
- Temporality of association (i.e. putative cause must antedate outcome of interest)
- Biological gradient (i.e. dose-response effect)
- Experimental evidence to support a causal association
- A plausible hypothesis to explain a causal association.

time to onset the illness in any given year, purely as an artefact of their month of birth. Despite these criticisms, it seems that there is a Northern hemisphere season-of-birth effect for schizophrenia, but the signal is very weak and the elevated risk very modest.

Maternal infection: An obvious question growing from the season-of-birth data is what exactly is it about those months that carry risk. The putative factor to come under closest scrutiny is maternal exposure to infectious agents, which may perturb foetal brain development at crucial stages and add to the risk of later schizophrenia. The 1957 influenza A2 pandemic provided an opportunity to test this hypothesis, given the steady and uniform progression of the virus across the globe. Studies from a number of countries, including Denmark and the United Kingdom, have shown an ecological association of increased schizophrenia births to women whose foetuses were in their second trimester of development during the pandemic. This effect seems to hold for influenza type A2, and has not been convincingly shown for other infectious disease pandemics, discounting a general effect due to maternal pyrexia, for example, or the effect of antipyretic drugs taken by the mother.

A more precise way of looking at this issue is to study the mother–child dyads directly. An opportunity to do this was afforded by the examination of maternal and cord blood samples in a number of North American birth cohorts. Elevated maternal cytokine levels (a marker of infection) were associated with later schizophrenia in the offspring, in a dose–response manner. Also, adult psychosis was more likely in the offspring of those mothers with elevated levels of IgG and IgM, and antibodies to Herpes simplex type 2. Again, causal pathways are complex and causality cannot be definitively concluded.

Maternal malnutrition: Another intriguing effect has been noted in the elevated risk of schizophrenia in foetuses in their first trimester of development during the Dutch Famine Winter, where the Northern part of Holland was subject to severe food rationing during the Nazi occupation. However, the fact that countries with pervasively poor maternal nutrition do not appear to have elevated rates of schizophrenia speak against this being a major universal effect. Having said this, certain nutritional factors might be specifically implicated here. Vitamin D, for example, has been forwarded as worthy of particular scrutiny on the basis of epidemiological findings such as the elevated risk of schizophrenia among the offspring of dark-skinned African-Caribbeans living in relatively sunlight-deprived climates (the United Kingdom), and rodent work showing effects of vitamin D deprivation on certain aspects of neurodevelopment.

Pregnancy and birth complications (PBCs): More broadly, complications of pregnancy and birth have been shown in a number of studies and several meta-analyses, to be associated with increased risk of schizophrenia in the offspring. This needs to be seen in the context that mothers with schizophrenia are in any event liable to experience PBCs (probably a complex effect due, *inter alia*, to maternal smoking, poor nutrition, and suboptimal neonatal care). The other factor is that a foetus with a neurodevelopmental disorder could be expected to be liable to PBCs, for example, through abnormal motor movements resulting in transverse lie or breech presentation: such effects have been shown for children with cerebral palsy.

Recently, researchers have suggested that *maternal stress* (in this case the death of a relative) during the first trimester of pregnancy is associated with a higher risk of schizophrenia occurring later on in that offspring. This is certainly intuitive, in the sense that expectant mothers are told that they should avoid stressful situations during the pregnancy, but it needs to be studied further. Also, several research groups have shown that the *older the father* is at time of conception, the greater the risk that this offspring will develop schizophrenia.

All of these are curious and intriguing associations. However, as individual causes for schizophrenia, their contribution is likely to be small. Again, whether their impact is higher when other risk factors (especially genetic risks) also coalesce is presently not well understood.

5.3 Can illicit substances cause schizophrenia?

Fascinating recent work has focussed on whether cannabis, the most widely used illicit substance in the world, might be causally implicated in schizophrenia. There is no doubt that cannabis can cause psychosis-like symptoms. Its psychoactive moiety, delta-9-tetrahydrocannabinol (THC), was synthesized in the 1960s and human experiments have shown that, through its action on cannabinoid CB1 receptors, it produces a fairly predictable range of symptoms.

What is also increasingly clear is that some individuals are particularly vulnerable to develop these effects on exposure to cannabis. Such individuals arguably have more 'psychosis-proneness' than most people, and THC tips them into psychosis more readily, as sugar would raise blood glucose levels in someone with glucose intolerance. There is some evidence that one marker of such proneness is carrying the Val-Val allele of the *COMT* gene (see Section 5.1).

It is obvious that people with schizophrenia have very marked 'psychosis-proneness', and it is thus no surprise that exposure to cannabis in such individuals is associated with a high likelihood of psychotic relapse. Indeed, cannabis use is one of the best predictors of a poor longitudinal course in people with schizophrenia, including more relapses and re-hospitalizations.

Whether cannabis can actually *cause* schizophrenia is, however, a rather different question, and one that should be considered with reference to Bradford-Hill's criteria for causality (see Box 5.3). The best study design to address the causality issue is the cohort study, as it is then clear that the exposure (cannabis) antedates the outcome (schizophrenia). A number of cohort studies, including the Swedish and Israeli conscript cohorts and the Dunedin and Christchurch birth cohorts from New Zealand, converge in the conclusion that teenage or young adult exposure to cannabis is associated with a small increased risk of later schizophrenia or schizophreniform psychosis, even after controlling for confounders such as urban dwelling, socio-economic status, marital status, gender, and ethnicity.

These studies suggest strongly that cannabis can be considered a (weak) causal factor in schizophrenia. But of course the vast majority of cannabis users do not develop schizophrenia, and the fact that rates of schizophrenia are fairly even across settings with very different rates of cannabis use speak against its being a major causal factor. Thus, cannabis needs to act in concert with other vulnerability factors to act as a cumulative causal factor in some cases of schizophrenia. An insight into this model is afforded by the Dunedin birth cohort, where an interaction was found between psychosis-like symptoms at age 11 and cannabis exposure at age 15 being associated with later schizophreniform psychosis.

5.4 **Are families to blame for schizophrenia?**

There have been a number of theories about causality in schizophrenia that have laid the onus of blame on families in general, or mothers in particular. For example, in the 1940s Fromm-Reichman, on the basis of a small number of observed cases, articulated the view that certain mothers were 'schizophrenogenic'. By this she meant that these mothers had an excess of psychological abnormalities and this could be tied to increased risk of schizophrenia in the offspring.

Lidz and colleagues looked more broadly at family dynamics, and reported two types of abnormal family pattern, which they labelled marital *skew* (one parent—usually the father—consistently yielded to the other's eccentricities) and marital *schism* (parents usually holding different views to each other, thus confusing the child). They suggested these patterns were causal rather than a consequence of schizophrenia in the offspring, but this has never been proven and has been abandoned as a causal theory.

Bateson in the 1950s analysed patterns of family communication in schizophrenia, and described 'double bind' where one form of instruction by a parent is contradicted by a less prominent but palpable conflicting instruction. For example, saying something nice and supportive, but in an angry and rejecting tone. And Singer and Wynne described 'amorphous' and 'fragmented' communication patterns in the parents of people with schizophrenia. Again, any causal role of these communication patterns has been discounted.

In many ways these sorts of theory were damaging to and blaming of families, and they have largely been abandoned. Our more modern view is that families can have a very important role to play in influencing the longitudinal course of the illness of their family member with schizophrenia, and should be given help and support to deal most effectively with the challenges related to this scenario. The reader is referred to Part 2 of this book for details of family interventions for schizophrenia.

Chapter 6

Schizophrenia as a brain disease

Key points

- There is good evidence that there are a range of structural brain changes associated with schizophrenia, though none are pathognomonic and the overlap with 'normal' is considerable.
- Functional brain imaging is helping us to better understand the brain processes underpinning the symptoms and deficits associated with schizophrenia.
- The neurodevelopmental model of schizophrenia has considerable heuristic appeal, though it cannot readily account for those patients with an onset of illness in middle or late life.
- The dopamine hypothesis of schizophrenia remains a very powerful explanatory model for many of the symptoms of schizophrenia, but serotonergic, glutamatergic, and other mechanisms are also implicated.

6.1 Is the brain abnormal in schizophrenia?

The answer to this question is both 'yes' and 'no'. Studies of brain structure have shown a tendency for the brains of people with schizophrenia to exhibit a range of differences from controls at an aggregate level; but all studied samples show considerable overlap with 'normal', and no study has demonstrated pathognomic brain changes in schizophrenia.

In fact, the idea that there are structural brain abnormalities in schizophrenia has a very long history, such that in one of the Victorian asylums, it was demonstrated that there was greater displacement of water from the ventricular system of post-mortem schizophrenia brains, compared to controls. But the fact that schizophrenia is a brain disease was largely forgotten, especially in the United States where psychodynamic influences pervaded psychiatry for decades.

The modern rediscovery of the brain in schizophrenia coincided with the then novel neuroimaging technique, computerized tomography (CT) scanning. Eve Johnstone, Tim Crow and colleagues at Northwick Park Hospital in London published, in 1976, a hugely important (and at the time hugely controversial) paper showing increased ventricular brain ratio (VBR) in people with schizophrenia. This finding has been demonstrated over and over, and a number of other findings have been fairly consistently shown using different neuroimaging techniques (see Box 6.1).

Thus, the extent and range of structural brain changes in schizophrenia are fairly well accepted. The emphasis of abnormality seems to be on the left hemisphere, compatible with the notion that schizophrenia is an essentially left hemisphere disorder, with an important impact on language. What is also fairly well accepted is that to some extent at least, these abnormalities antedate the onset of illness, being demonstrable in first episode samples. This has been referred to as a 'static encephalopathy', a notion consistent with the neurodevelopmental model (see Section 6.4). Recently, however, Christos Pantelis and colleagues in Melbourne, Australia, showed that 'preschizophrenic' individuals at high risk for the illness show progressive brain structural changes in the period before the evolution of frank psychotic symptoms. Whether this is a marker of innate abnormalities in synaptic pruning and other developmental changes, or is consequent upon the prepsychotic process itself, is not yet clear.

Another contentious issue is whether the brain continues to change over the longitudinal course of the illness. Lyn DeLisi in New York, for example, performed an important follow-up study of young people with schizophrenia, with serial neuroimaging, and reported progressive changes in some cortical areas. These findings have been replicated by other investigators, and consensus seems to be that there are ongoing brain changes which act 'on top of' the static encephalopathy.

Box 6.1 Structural brain abnormalities in schizophrenia

General

- Enlarged lateral ventricles
- Enlarged third ventricle
- Reduced overall grey matter volume
- Widespread cortical and cerebellar atrophy.

Site-specific

- *Frontal lobe*: volume reduction, especially inferior prefrontal cortex
- *Temporal lobe:* volume reduction in amygdala, hippocampus, parahippocampal gyrus; appears more marked on left side.

First episode studies have also suggested that these progressive changes are more pronounced in patients with a poor illness outcome, compared to those with a more benign longitudinal course. Whether adequate treatment can ameliorate these progressive changes is controversial. The longitudinal first episode study of Jeff Lieberman and colleagues has provided evidence that patients on haloperidol showed progressive brain structural abnormalities to a degree not seen in those treated with olanzapine. This finding has led to the hypothesis that the atypical antipsychotics are 'neuroprotective': clearly more work needs to be done to confirm or refute this.

6.2 What have we learnt from functional brain imaging?

As is described in Section 6.6, abnormal dopamine chemistry (either too much, too little, unstable, or dysregulated) has been a central theme in trying to understand schizophrenia. This has been particularly so in trying to understand how antipsychotic medications might work in the brain. However, these dopamine changes and their relationship to treatment have been hard to prove until the advent of several functional brain imaging techniques (summarized in Box 6.2).

Laurelle and colleagues broke new ground in a positron emission tomography (PET) study when they showed that there was an excess of dopamine in the brains of patients who had just become psychotic (and had never received medications) and that this overactivity was also directly proportional to just how psychotic the patients were at the time of scanning. Others have replicated this key observation.

Conversely, others have used PET to study the prefrontal cortex of the brain where it is believed that underactivity of dopamine contributes to many of the negative symptoms of schizophrenia. They have shown that there is underactivity in metabolism in this key region, especially in patients who have prominent negative symptoms ('deficit syndrome') as part of their illness. As mentioned earlier, Peter Liddle and others have tried to 'map' distinct symptom domains to particular brain regions (see Box 2.3). Also, Philip McGuire and colleagues in London have conducted a series of fascinating studies (using functional Magnetic Resonance Imaging (fMRI)) that simply ask

---

Box 6.2 Types of functional brain imaging techniques

- Positron Emission Tomography (PET)
- Single Photon Emission Tomography (SPECT)
- Functional Magnetic Resonance Imaging (fMRI)
- Magnetic Resonance Spectroscopy (MRS).

the question, 'Which regions of the brain are active when patients hear voices?' They have pretty convincingly localized this effect to the temporal cortex, and proposed that this area gets 'excited' on its own (i.e. the cells fire off without any external stimulus), and the person then experiences this as 'hearing voices' as if they came from outside his/her head.

Although all of this work is really interesting and is much liked by phenomenologists (researchers and clinicians who meticulously study patients' symptoms), the idea of symptom maps is probably too simple. Other researchers favour the notion that symptoms (perhaps especially thought disorder) arise from a fundamental dysconnectivity of brain 'hard-wiring' in schizophrenia, associated with an overall 'chaotic' pattern of functional imaging brain abnormalities.

Functional brain imaging (chiefly PET and its sister technique SPECT) has also been helpful in furthering our understanding of how antipsychotic medications work (see also Part 2 of this book). In a series of elegant studies, Kapur and colleagues in Toronto showed that the drugs had to bind to dopamine receptors at a minimal rate of 60% occupancy in order to work. The problem for the first-generation typical antipsychotics was that they easily overshot that occupancy rate and once a 75–80% rate is reached, the drugs cause extrapyramidal side effects (EPSEs). This pattern is more complex with second-generation antipsychotics. For instance, it appears that olanzapine, ziprasidone, and (to a lesser extent) risperidone are partly buffered from this effect—possibly because they also bind strongly to serotonin receptors. Clozapine and quetiapine appear to have different receptor profiles altogether, in that they never (no matter how much drug is given) seem to hit that magic 60% occupancy rate—and yet they clearly are effective in treating schizophrenia.

As neuroimaging capability has advanced, it has become possible to study other neurotransmitters that are considered important in schizophrenia. For example, magnetic resonance spectroscopy (MRS) studies have shown reductions in glutamate levels and glutamine in schizophrenia patients. Also, MRS has revealed reductions in N-acetyl-aspartate levels (NAA) that is thought to reflect damage/ impaired functioning/loss of brain cells. These theories are expanded upon later in this chapter.

6.3 Is there a neuropathology of schizophrenia?

The neurosurgeon Fred Plum famously called schizophrenia the 'graveyard' of neuropathologists, alluding to the lack of consistent findings in the field. What has been a consistent finding, though, has been the lack of gliosis (scar tissue) in the brains of people with schizophrenia. This suggests that any insult that occurred early in brain development (before the third trimester), was before the brain was capable of producing a gliotic response.

Post-mortem studies have also shown neuronal disarray in hippocampus and entorhinal cortex, and decreased size of thalamic neurons. Evidence has also been produced for increased neuronal density (suggesting a reduction in dendrites) in dorsolateral prefrontal cortex, compatible with the hypofrontality demonstrated on functional neuroimaging, and findings of reduction in the neuronal marker NAA (see Section 6.2).

6.4 Is there a consistent neurophysiology of schizophrenia?

The schizophrenia field has adopted a number of neurophysiologic techniques to explore neuropsychological theories of the disorder and/ or to describe enophenotypes for schizophrenia. The main modalities in use are outlined in Box 6.3.

It has long been shown that there are *eye tracking abnormalities* in patients with schizophrenia. Since these (and deficits in other physiological measures) are also seen in the 'healthy' relatives of patients with schizophrenia (although they are much less prominent), researchers have considered these abnormalities as possible biomarkers of the heritability of schizophrenia. In other words, they might be signs of an underlying vulnerability to schizophrenia and thereby be expressed in those at potential risk to develop the condition (e.g. people in their prodrome of schizophrenia or children of parents who have schizophrenia) or be carried by otherwise healthy parents.

Thus, eye tracking deficits, along with auditory P300 abnormalities, mismatch negativity, and sensory gating abnormalities may potentially be used to define what are called 'endophenotypes' of schizophrenia. Researchers have also used this approach to try to tease out the genetic contributions to schizophrenia. Also, sensory gating deficits (e.g. delays in P450 sensory stimulus activity) are often proposed to explain schizophrenia as a disorder where the brain gets 'overloaded'. In these theories, the sensory gating mechanism (a kind of

---

Box 6.3 Neurophysiologic techniques employed in schizophrenia

- Eye tracking
- P300 and P450 event-related potentials
- Mismatch negativity
- Sensory gating abnormalities.

'sunscreen' for the brain that protects it from overexposure to sensory inputs from the environment) is defective and so the patient is barraged by external stimuli, resulting in confusion and uncertainty about what comes from within (e.g. internal thoughts) and what comes from outside (e.g. perceptual disturbances). Similar to many theories about schizophrenia, the sensory gating mechanism is elegant but probably overly simplistic.

6.5 Is the neurodevelopmental model parsimonious?

A major contribution to our thinking about schizophrenia has been the explicit expostulation of the neurodevelopmental model by researchers in the United States (Daniel Weinberger and colleagues) and the United Kingdom (Robin Murray and co-workers at London's Institute of Psychiatry). The notion is that schizophrenia has its roots in aberrant development of the brain, but that the illness only manifests with positive symptoms in late teens/early adulthood when the brain develops the capacity to produce such symptoms. The neurodevelopmental model appropriately encompasses genetic and non-genetic aetiological factors, operating in concert with cumulative causal factors in any individual.

It would seem that a genetic predisposition is vital, as it sets the backdrop upon which other factors can impact neurodevelopment at key stages. As Peter Jones and Robin Murray stated, 'the genetics of schizophrenia is (sic) the genetics of neurodevelopment'. The implication of neurodevelopmental genes such as neuregulin and dysbindin and DISC1 in the aetiology of schizophrenia (see Section 5.1) reinforce this notion, as do findings that it is the early-onset neurodevelopmental type of illness that carries the greatest familial loading for schizophrenia.

Another pointer towards the neurodevelopmental origins of schizophrenia lies in subtle morphological variants that reflect early ectodermal development and purportedly mirror neurodevelopment. Thus, people with schizophrenia are more likely to exhibit a number of features, including high-arched palate, low-set ears, and widely spaced eyes. They are also more likely to show abnormalities in the development of finger whorls, with unusual dermatoglyphic patterns. Of course such markers are non-specific and are shared by many people without schizophrenia, but do seem to provide evidence of early developmental deviance in some cases of schizophrenia. Of interest is that such markers are more common in the affected twin of monozygotic twin pairs discordant for schizophrenia, consonant with the fact that the affected twin is more likely to exhibit structural brain abnormalities, compared to the well co-twin.

A neurodevelopmental subtype of schizophrenia has been offered support from latent class analysis of the Camberwell Register cohort. This subtype is characterized by an early onset (mostly below 25 years), male preponderance, poor premorbid development, negative symptoms, and genetic and early environmental risk factors (notably pregnancy and birth complications). It will not go unnoticed that this proposed subtype resonates well with Kraepelin's description of dementia praecox; a poor longitudinal trajectory is implicit.

But, as David Castle and Robin Murray point out, this model leaves unaccounted for later onset 'milder' forms of the illness. Of course such later onset cases might also have neurodevelopmental loadings, but their better premorbid and longitudinal course and the fact they onset after the bulk of brain development has occurred suggest that other factors are operating. One putative factor is the withdrawal of oestrogens in women at menopause, though any such effect has not been convincingly demonstrated at anything other than the aggregate level. Oestrogen withdrawal also cannot readily be implicated in those cases with an onset in very late life, in whom neurodegenerative influences of various kinds might be important.

6.6 What is the neurochemistry of schizophrenia?

Dopaminergic mechanisms: Traditionally, neurochemical explanations for schizophrenia have emphasized the centrality of perturbation of dopaminergic systems (see Figure 6.1). This model was based on a number of observations, notably that substances such as amphetamines cause dopamine release and hence cause psychotic symptoms and that medications that block dopamine D2 receptors ameliorate such symptoms (see Box 6.4).

But, of course, schizophrenia is not just about positive symptoms and many other disorders are associated with delusions and hallucinations. A twist to the dopamine hypothesis, then, is that whilst positive symptoms might be due to a hyperdopaminergic state in mesolimbic tracts, negative symptoms are thought to be due to hypodopaminergia in mesocortical tracts. This view gains support from the fact that typical antipsychotics that block dopamine D2 receptors fairly indiscriminately can result in a worsening of negative symptoms (the so-called neurolept-induced deficit syndrome, or NIDS).

But the dopamine hypothesis has not gained much support from neuroimaging studies. For example, there is little consistency in findings of abnormalities of D2 receptor binding in the brains of people with schizophrenia. Also, early reports of abnormalities in cerebrospinal fluid levels of breakdown products of dopamine in schizophrenia have not been consistently replicated.

Figure 6.1 Brain dopamine pathways, perturbations in schizophrenia and in response to dopamine D2 receptor antagonism

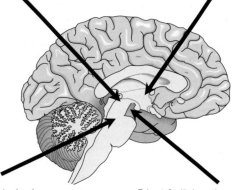

Mesolimbic pathway
- Relative excess of DA → positive symptoms

Mesocortical pathway
- Relative paucity of DA → negative & cognitive symptoms
- DA blockade worsens negative symptoms

Nigostriatal pathway
- DA blockade → dystonias
                → Parkinsonism
                → dyskinesias
                → akathisia

Tuberoinfundibular pathway
- DA blockade → hyper-prolactinaemia

DA = dopamine antagonism

Box 6.4 Underpinnings of the dopamine hypothesis of schizophrenia

- Medications that are dopamine antagonists ameliorate positive symptoms of psychosis, and their potency is directly correlated with their tenacity for dopamine D2 receptors.
- Amphetamines and other agents which cause dopamine release in the brain can cause psychotic symptoms.
- Amphetamine exposure results in more marked dopamine release in people with schizophrenia than non-schizophrenia controls.
- Dopaminergic agents can cause delusions and hallucinations.
- Disulfiram, which inhibits dopamine hydroxylase, can exacerbate schizophrenic symptoms.

Furthermore, the limitations of the dopamine hypothesis are evident at a clinical level from the failure of response of some 30% of schizophrenia patients to blockade of over 60% of dopamine D2 receptors with typical antipsychotic agents; and the clear advantage of clozapine (a complex agent that has pharmacological activity across a range of brain systems) as a therapeutic agent in some of these 'treatment resistant' patients.

Serotonergic mechanisms: It has long been recognized that the serotonergic agonist lysergic acid diethylamide (LSD) is an hallucinogen, but interest in the role of serotonergic mechanisms in schizophrenia was spurred by the observation that the first 'atypical' antipsychotic, clozapine, binds to serotonin 5HT-2A receptors. Herb Meltzer advocated that it was the ratio of 5HT-2A:dopamine D2 blockade that gave clozapine its unique advantage over typical agents in its very low propensity to cause EPSEs; serotonergic and dopaminergic pathways interact reciprocally in nigrostriatal pathways.

This notion led, *inter alia*, to the development of a number of novel atypical antipsychotics, all of which (except for amisulpride, the 'atypical atypical'), to some degree, emulate this pharmacological property of clozapine. These agents include risperidone, paliperidone, olanzapine, quetiapine, ziprasidone, aripiprazole, and sertindole. However, all these agents have other pharmacodynamic actions, including muscarinic (M1), histaminergic (H1), and alpha-adrenergic receptor blockade (for details see Chapter 8).

Furthermore, neuroimaging studies have failed consistently to show abnormalities in 5HT-2A receptor binding in the brain of people with schizophrenia, or in cerebrospinal fluid levels of 5-hydroxyindole acetic acid (5-H1AA), the major breakdown product of 5-HT. Also, there is no evidence that serotonergic antagonists are of themselves antipsychotic. Thus, the serotonin hypothesis gains most support from observations of interactions with the dopamine system.

Glutamatergic mechanisms: Phencyclidine (PCP), an antagonist of the *N*-methyl-D-aspartate (NMDA) subtype of the glutamatergic receptor, can produce a clinical picture that looks much like schizophrenia. This and other observations, including the fact that ketamine (another NMDA receptor antagonist) causes more marked psychotic symptoms in people with schizophrenia than in controls with no mental illness, have given substance to a glutamate hypothesis of schizophrenia. Recent findings that a selective metabotropic glutamate 2/3 agonist can reduce positive and negative symptoms of schizophrenia have opened up a potential new therapeutic avenue for this disorder. Actually, glutamate is a modifier of a number of different neurotransmitters, including dopamine, so certainly this does not obviate the importance of dopamine in the pathogenesis of schizophrenia.

Muscarinic mechanisms: Both clozapine and olanzapine (and to a lesser extent quetiapine) show affinity for muscarinic-M1 receptors. Thus, some researchers have been drawn to the muscarinic system in the quest for new treatments for schizophrenia. Work in this area has still to develop.

Cannabinoid mechanisms: The psychomimetic action of delta-9-tetrahydrocannabinol (THC) and the associations between THC use and schizophrenia have been detailed earlier. Of interest is that, although THC acts via cannabinoid CB1 receptors to produce its psychomimetic effects, the CB1 receptor antagonist rimonabant does not appear to have efficacy in the treatment of schizophrenia. However, an enhanced understanding of the cannabinoid system might inform treatments for this disorder. Intriguingly, for example, tetra-hydrocannabidiol might have antipsychotic efficacy.

Part 2

Treatments

Chapter 7

Models of care

Key points

- The optimal treatment of a person with schizophrenia requires a coherent and consistent longitudinal plan.
- Patient education and empowerment is a key part of helping them stay well.
- The stress–strengths–vulnerability approach has considerable appeal in the management of schizophrenia.
- Moves to community care of people with schizophrenia has restricted but not obviated the role of acute inpatient facilities.

7.1 How is it best to approach the treatment of someone with schizophrenia?

The general principles underpinning the treatment of schizophrenia must include a comprehensive longitudinal approach, relevant to the illness stage, tailored to the individual, and encompassing biological, psychological, and social domains. It should also be cognizant of the context in which the individual lives, including family, work, and accommodation.

To achieve this, a multidisciplinary team is usually required, with each professional within the team bringing their own expertise to bear, but with a coordinator who can ensure consistency and comprehensiveness of interventions. In many countries, this latter role is filled by a case manager, who also helps guide the patient in negotiating the complexities of service delivery systems.

There is a strong current vogue to cement plans for people with schizophrenia, to include them actively in this process, and to monitor outcomes on a regular basis. This planning includes ongoing assessment of risk, including to self or others but more broadly also to do with elements such as self-neglect, substance use, and physical health issues. This can be a very constructive process, allowing all involved to reflect on priorities for the individual (e.g. getting a job, ensuring physical health is optimized); to assess what has helped in the past and what has been less helpful; to agree and document warning signs of relapse; and to set in place plans for when such signs recur.

There are a number of structured approaches which can allow this process to occur. *The strengths model*, for example, focuses on the person's abilities rather than on the disabilities or symptoms. Concrete goals are set to achieve meaningful life activities. Treating symptoms becomes a secondary, albeit still necessary, goal. This approach has developed further under the *consumerism/recovery model*, such that patients (often referred to then as 'clients') become much more active in deciding about their care and in goal setting. Another extension of this recovery model is the use of peer supports, that is, people who have mental illness who can lend a 'helping hand' in the patient's recovery. This is rather similar to the 'sponsor' model of Alcoholics Anonymous.

Collaborative therapy is an Australian model which places the individual at the centre of care and empowers him/her with the skills necessary to live with his/her illness in a positive manner. Using a modified stress–strengths–vulnerability process, it is in many aspects a chronic disease model and uses a small pocket diary (a collaborative treatment journal, or CTJ), *inter alia*: to record early warning signs and relapse prevention plans; to map collaborative partners who can assist them; and to allow practice of relapse prevention strategies.

Personal therapy (PT) was developed by Gerry Hogarty and colleagues in the United States. This approach 'drilled down' on the particular strengths and relapse risk pattern for each individual patient and was greeted with great enthusiasm. Unfortunately, it never gained hold both because it was (too) labour intensive and, because sadly, the inventor Dr Hogarty died shortly after the first series of studies were published.

Assertive community treatment, also known as intensive case management, is a well-established intensive model for assisting people with more severe forms of schizophrenia, and who carry a number of disabilities. Often referred to as the 'revolving door' patients, these individuals can benefit greatly from the continuity of care and high frequency of clinical contacts that this model can offer, with improvements in control of illness and a reduction in hospitalizations. But to work it does need to meet fidelity requirements, as shown in Box 7.1. High-profile, recent UK studies have failed to meet these fidelity requirements, and have thus not demonstrated any benefit for individuals.

> **Box 7.1 Components of an assertive community outreach team**
> - Low case loads (usually < 10 patients per case manager)
> - A multidisciplinary team
> - Ability to deliver care in the community
> - Ability to provide long-term continuity of care
> - High level of face-to-face contact (at least twice a week, and up to twice daily, if required)
> - Assertive follow-up
> - 24hr/7-day cover optimally
> - Service provided from within team mostly, but able to liaise with other services as necessary.

7.2 What is the place of inpatient care for people with schizophrenia?

In countries that have embraced community care, there has been a massive shift of staff, resources, and patients from stand-alone psychiatric hospitals into the community. This has left the provision of inpatient care, once the major care setting for people with severe mental illness, in a much restricted role. Regrettably, some of the positive attributes of the old 'asylums' (e.g. group-based therapies, vocational training) have been threatened, and there is a risk that inpatient care will become little more than a setting for containment of acute risk.

Acute inpatient care is still a vital component of modern psychiatric services, at the very least for the short-term management of people in crisis, who have suffered a relapse of illness, and/or who cannot be safely managed in the community. Many modern inpatient units are co-located with general hospitals, have very high turnover and occupancy rates, and a short duration of stay. These units tend to deal with patients whose symptoms are very florid, and who may be at risk of harm to self or others. Rates of aggression and assault are often high, and it is crucial that such units have well-developed regimes for dealing with acute psychiatric emergencies (see Chapter 10).

Despite these pressures, much useful work can be done in inpatient settings, including psychosocial interventions. Admission to hospital can afford an opportunity for a full and detailed review of the patient and their management, and allow the setting of clear interdisciplinary longer-term plans. It is important that these plans are agreed with the patient and their usual community-based treatment team. Other uses of inpatient care are shown in Box 7.2.

Box 7.2 Uses of acute inpatient psychiatric facilities

- Provision of a safe environment
- Physical health review
- Multidisciplinary review and formulation
- Management of psychiatric symptoms, including optimal psychopharmacology
- Psychoeducation
- Teaching coping skills
- Family involvement
- Longer-term planning, including relapse prevention strategies.

Longer-term inpatient facilities are a very useful adjunct to acute units. Optimally, they should be based in the community and provide as close to a 'normal' living environment as possible. Facilities should be provided to enable upskilling in areas such as shopping, budgeting, cooking, and cleaning. Levels of staff support vary according to needs, such that some units have full-time clinical cover with trained clinical staff, whilst others are run by non-government organizations using non-clinical staff but with clinical back-up from the local mental health service.

Chapter 8

Pharmacological and physical treatments

Key points

- Antipsychotic medication revolutionized the care of people with schizophrenia, and remains the mainstay of management.
- The newer atypical antipsychotics overall have advantages over the older typical agents, notably in terms of a lower propensity to extrapyramidal side effects (EPSEs).
- The 'atypicals' are not a class, and each agent should be considered on its potential efficacy and side effect profile for each individual patient.
- A number of atypicals have a problematic side effect profile, notably in terms of physical health risks; these need to be routinely monitored and managed.
- Clozapine remains the most effective of the antipsychotics, but its risk profile is such that it should generally be reserved for patients who have failed to respond adequately to at least two other antipsychotic agents.
- Negative and cognitive symptoms respond less well to antipsychotics than do positive symptoms, though various adjunctive medication and non-medication strategies may benefit individual patients.

There is no doubt that medication plays a crucial role in the acute and maintenance treatment of schizophrenia. The discovery of chlorpromazine in the 1950s heralded a new era in the treatment of this disorder, and arguably allowed the deinstitutionalization process to occur. But the older antipsychotics carry a burden of side effects, notably through their impact on the extrapyramidal nervous system, which left the field searching for effective antipsychotics which did not have these detrimental effects. The relatively recent advent of 'atypical' antipsychotic medications was much vaunted as a breakthrough in this regard, and these agents have largely supplanted the older 'typicals' in many parts of the world. But some sceptics still question whether they are really better. Also, they often tend to be lumped together as a 'class' whereas they are really an array of agents with different pharmacokinetic and pharmacodynamic properties, and different side effect profiles.

8.1 Are atypical antipsychotics really better than the older drugs and are they different from each other?

The atypical antipsychotics are shown in Box 8.1. There is no compelling evidence that the newer atypical agents (i.e. excepting clozapine) are more effective at treating the psychotic symptoms associated with schizophrenia. Meta-analytic studies pooling the main randomized controlled trials of the atypicals have concluded that they are no better than the older agents in terms of efficacy against positive symptoms. The first phase of the landmark Clinical Antipsychotic Trials of Intervention Effectiveness (CATIE) trials in the United States found that all-cause discontinuation rates for a range of atypical agents (apart from olanzapine) were no more favourable than for the typical agent perphenazine. And the Cost Utility of the Latest Antipsychotic Drugs in Schizophrenia Studies (CUtLASS) in Europe found broadly comparable overall outcomes for typicals and atypicals.

However, the effectiveness of any intervention in schizophrenia needs to be assessed across multiple domains, and include longer-term side effect risk. What does seem to be the case is that, in general, atypicals at least do not make negative and cognitive symptoms worse (and some may have positive effects with respect to these domains: see Section 8.8). And what is beyond doubt is that they carry a lower burden of EPSEs at usual therapeutic doses. Disfiguring and stigmatizing tardive dyskinesia, in particular, appears to be much rarer than with the typical antipsychotics.

As mentioned earlier, the atypicals are not a single class of agents, and we do not yet have a way of knowing which will work for whom, and what side effects will prove problematic. However, in clinical practice an 'informed guess' as to the most suitable agent for an individual patient can be guided by knowledge of prior response and tolerability in that individual, and/or reference to the clinical tips shown in Table 8.1. It is hoped that in future pharmacogenomic analyses will allow us to predict individual responsivity and propensity to side effects better.

Clozapine bears particular mention, as it still stands apart from the other atypicals. The oldest of the atypicals, and in many ways the prototype, it has proven its worth in numerous clinical trials and has an established place in the treatment of patients who do not respond adequately to other agents. It does not cause EPSEs and is effective for both positive and negative symptoms, as well as in improving some aspects of cognition. However, it has a number of side effects, some of which are potentially lethal (see Table 8.1), and in most countries it is reserved for patients in whom other agents have failed or have produced intolerable side effects. Strict haematological monitoring is required, as described in Table 8.1, and many centres have mandated cardiac monitoring as well.

Table 8.1 Clinical tips about the atypical antipsychotics			
Agent	Usual daily clinical dose	Positive attributes	Potential negative attributes
Amisulpride	400–1200mg	• Effective for deficit syndrome at ≤300mg/d • No anticholineric or histaminergic activity	• Higher dose → emergent EPSE • Hyperprolactinaemia
Aripiprazole	10–30mg	• Low rate of Parkinsonism/dystonia • No hyperprolactinaemia • Negligible weight gain/metabolic problems	• Initial akathisia can be bothersome
Clozapine	200–900mg	• Proven efficacy in 'treatment resistance' • Negligible EPSE or TD	• Weight gain • Hyperlipidaemia • Emergent diabetes • Constipation • Sialorrohoea • Neutropaenia—requires blood monitoring • Cardiovascular problems
Olanzapine	5–20mg	• Effective for psychotic symptoms • Mood-stabilizing properties • Low propensity to EPSE • Tablet, dissolvable and short-acting parenteral forms	• Weight gain • Hyperlipidaemia • Emergent diabetes • Sedation can be bothersome in longer term

Table 8.1 (Contd.)			
Agent	Usual daily clinical dose	Positive attributes	Potential negative attributes
Paliperidone	3–12mg	• Slow release formulation means 'flat' dose–response curve • Long half-life • No up-titration required • Renal metabolism precludes most drug–drug interactions	• Higher doses might be associated with emergent EPSE and hyper-prolactinaemia
Quetiapine	300–750mg	• Wide dose range • Sedation can be helpful • Antidepressant and mood stabilizing effects • Very low EPSE • Can dose-titrate rapidly, especially with slow-release preparations	• Sedation can be problematic in longer term • Can be difficult to establish optimal dose • Weight gain • No parenteral formulation
Risperidone	4–6mg	• Effective for psychotic symptoms • Oral tablets and dissolvable forms • Long-acting injectible avaliable	• Postural hypo-tension if dose increased too rapidly • Emergent EPSE at higher doses • Hyperprolactinaemia
Sertindole	12–20mg	• Effective for positive and negative symptoms • Low rates of EPSE • Not sedating • No increase in prolactin	• Cardiac monitoring required
Ziprasidone	40—160mg	• Negligible weight gain/metabolic problems	• Prolongation of QTc • Can be sedating

* Information given in this table is for guidance only, please refer to your local regulatory and pharmaceutical sources for specifics on medication availability, dosage, and prescribing information.

8.2 What are the main side effects of the antipsychotics?

Extrapyramidal side effects (EPSEs): As outlined above, the older typical antipsychotics had as their main concerning set of side effects those consequent upon dopamine D2 receptor blockade in the extrapyramidal system; these effects are collectively referred to as extrapyramidal side effects or EPSEs, and are summarized in Table 8.2.

Over 80% receptor occupancy has been shown on neuroimaging studies to be the threshold at which these EPSEs manifest, and as around 60% occupancy is required for antipsychotic efficacy, the 'therapeutic window' is narrow.

'Atypicality' is variously defined, but the most common clinical use is to refer to those antipsychotics that, at usual antipsychotic doses, do not cause EPSEs. This definition is problematic in that some 'typical' agents (e.g. the phenothiazines) have a relatively low propensity for ESPEs, whilst some 'atypicals' (e.g. risperidone, amisulpride) actually do cause EPSEs at higher doses in some people.

Tardive dyskinesia (TD) is a particularly problematic side effect which is well described in association with longer-term use of typical

Table 8.2 Extrapyramidal side effects (EPSEs) of antipsychotics, and their treatment

		Signs and symptoms	Treatment
Parkinsonism		• Cogwheel rigidity • Shuffling gait with restricted arm swing • Restriction of effect ('mask-like' facies)	• Lower dose of antipsychotic • Use atypical anti-psychotic • Anticholinergic agent
Dystonias	*Acute*	• Opisthotonos • Laryngeal dystonia (can be fatal)	• Immediate treatment with anticholinergic (can use IMI or IVI if required)
	Tardive	• E.g. 'postural' abnormality with 'limping' gait due to paraspinal muscle dystonia	• Lower dose • Use atypical agent • Anticholinergic agent
Dyskinesias	*Acute*		• Lower dose or change antipsychotic
	Tardive	• Orofaciobuccolingual • Truncal and limb dyskinesias	• Complex: see p. 66

Akathisia		• Observed motor restlessness
		• Subjective 'need to move', especially legs
			• Lower dose of antipsychotic
			• Use atypical anti-psychotic
			• Cover with short term
			  • beta-blocker
			  • benzodiazepine
			  • clonidine

antipsychotics, and thought to be a consequence of hypersensitization of dopamine receptors. It is characterized by oro-facio-bucco-lingual movements, which can become grotesque and even interfere with speaking and swallowing; associated limb dyskinesias may also be present. The risk appears much lower with the atypicals, although arguably only clozapine has been on the market long enough to be sure this advantage holds up over decades of treatment. Other risks factors for TD are shown in Box 8.1.

Treatment of TD is tricky. Simply withdrawing the antipsychotic can actually make the movements worse, though instituting an atypical (notably clozapine) can be beneficial in the longer term. Withdrawal of any anticholinergic medication is also suggested, though again initially the movement disorder may worsen. Other strategies include the addition to the antipsychotic of vitamin E, nifedipine, clonidine, clonazepam, or reserpine. Each agent should be tried sequentially, and efficacy and side effects evaluated over a 3-month period before moving on to the next choice.

Neuroleptic malignant syndrome (NMS) is a rare but potentially fatal side effect. The main features are shown in Box 8.2. NMS is more common with high doses of parenteral typical antipsychotics administered over a short time period in a highly aroused patient, but has also been described with most of the atypicals. Treatment is largely medical, with appropriate supportive care (often intensive care is required), immediate cessation of the offending antipsychotic, and administration of bromocriptine and/or dantrolene. Re-exposure to an antipsychotic needs to be performed judiciously, with appropriate clinical monitoring; an atypical agent is much preferred.

Box 8.1 Risk factors for tardive dyskinesia

- Advancing age (definitely)
- Female gender (probably)
- Long exposure to high doses of antipsychotics (expressly typicals)
- Affective features (equivocal).

Box 8.2 Features of neuroleptic malignant syndrome (NMS)

- Muscle rigidity
- Pyrexia
- Autonomic instability
- Altered consciousness
- Elevated white cell count
- Markedly elevated creatine phosphokinase level.

Metabolic issues: Weight gain, diabetes, hyperlipidaemia, and the metabolic syndrome have been discussed earlier. They are more common with some agents than others, and are a major contributor to cardiovascular risk. Thus, monitoring and appropriate treatments are crucial, as discussed below (see Figure 8.1 for a monitoring proforma).

Cardiac side effects: Many of the antispychotics can cause transient tachycardia, perhaps most prominent with clozapine. Postural hypotension can occur with those agents that block alpha-1-adrenergic receptors (e.g. risperidone), and care should be taken if up-titrating such agents rapidly. Clozapine has been associated with a very rare (perhaps 1 in 1000 risk) fulminant myocarditis, with a 40% fatality rate; and a less rare but less dangerous and more indolent cardiomyopathy. Precautions to be taken are outlined below.

Prolongation of the QTc interval has been a focus of concern for some antipsychotics. The usual QTc is <420msec for males and <430msec for females. Concern regarding torsades de points and ventricular fibrillation arises as QTc intervals approach 500msec. Typical antipsychotics associated with concerning QTc prolongation include thioridazine, pimozide, and droperidol. Of the atypicals, ziprasidone and sertindole show greater propensity to QTc prolongation than the others, though post-marketing surveillance has not found these agents to be associated with increased cardiac death rates. It would seem sensible that in patients in whom such medications are being considered, a baseline and follow-up QTc and potassium and magnesium are performed.

Hyperprolactinaemia is a fairly common side effect of the typical antipsychotics, and of risperidone and amisulpride. It can be associated with menstrual irregularities and sexual dysfunction, and cause gynaecomastia and galactorrhoea (seemingly most common in young females). There are concerns about effects on bone mineral density, with a potential long-term risk of osteoporosis, especially in elderly women.

Other side effects of antipsychotics are shown in Box 8.3. The risk varies across agents and across individuals.

8.3 How is it best to go about switching antipsychotics?

The decision to switch antipsychotics is a complex one that should encompass a full review of the efficacy and side effects associated with the current agent, as well as prior agents. It requires an open discussion with the patient and (where appropriate) family members. The rationale and risks and benefits of the switch need to be articulated, and a plan put in place to manage the switch.

Figure 8.1 Metabolic monitoring proforma

SÌV	UR No.:
ST VINCENT'S MENTAL HEALTH	Surname:
METABOLIC MONITORING	Given Name:
	D.O.B.:
	Please ☐ in if no Patient Label available

INSTRUCTIONS FOR USE:
- *This form should be used for all patients on antipsychotics or mood stabilisers. It is suggested pertinent positive or negative results are documented in the boxes.*
- *Clozapine: This form is to be used only after the first 18 weeks.*
- *An authorised signed entry to be completed in the medical record progress notes for each measure on each occasion.*
- *Filing: this form should be filed in the Mental Health forms section of the record in order of most recent date of entry.*

Rapid No.		Base Date	3 Months	6 Months	12 Months	18 Months	24 Months	30 Months	36 Months
INSERT RESULT IN EACH CELL		..../..../....	..../..../....	..../..../....	..../..../....	..../..../....	..../..../....	..../..../....	..../..../....
Metabolic (for all patients on antipsychotics and mood stabilisers)	Height								
	Weight (in kg)								
	BMI = weight in kg by height in m2								
	Waist								
	Blood Pressure								
	Fasting Blood Glucose								
	Lipids (Chol, LDL, HDL, TG)								
	LFT								
	U&E								
	TFT								
Lithium	Lithium Level								
	FBE								
Sodium Valproate	Valproate Level								
	FBE								
Carbamazepine	Carbamazepine Level								
Clozapine Note: FBE as per Clozapine protocol	ECG								
	Echocardiogram								
	Troponin I/CK								
	Clozapine Level								
Prolactin elevating antipsychotics	Prolactin Level								
For patients on QTc prolonging antipsychotics	ECG								
Print name & signature of doctor completing this collection occasion:									

SV 654

ST VINCENT'S MENTAL HEALTH – METABOLIC MONITORING FORM

Box 8.3 Side effects of antipsychotics

- *Extrapyramidal effects* (worse with typical agents; least with clozapine): acute or chronic dystonias, dyskinesias, parkinsonism, akathisia (initial akathisia common with aripiprazole)
- *Anticholinergic:* dry mouth, constipation, blurring of vision (particular precaution in narrow-angle glaucoma), urinary hesitancy/retention (expressly males with enlarged prostate)
- *Cardiac effects:* transient (and sometimes enduring) tachycardia; postural hypotension (common in agents with alpha-1-adrenergic blockade); prolonged QTc interval (notably thioridazine, droperidol, ziprasidone, sertindole); myocarditis and cardiomyopathy (rare; risk appears higher with clozapine)
- *Sedation* (mostly related to histaminergic effects)
- *Lowered seizure threshold* (notably clozapine)
- *Prolactin elevation* (notably typicals, risperidone, amisulpride)
- *Weight gain, emergent diabetes, hypercholesterolaemia* (worst with clozapine and olanzapine; minimal with aripiprazole, ziprasidone)
- *Blood dyscrasias:* transient effects not uncommon with many agents; severe neutropaenia occurs in around 1 in 200 people taking clozapine; decreased platelet aggregation can occur, especially in conjunction with agents such as serotonergic antidepressants
- *Hepatic dysfunction:* transient elevation in some hepatic enzymes not uncommon; occasional more severe hepatitis (e.g. with chlorpromazine)
- *Skin:* photosensitivity common with chlorpromazine; other skin effects rare and idiosyncratic
- *Eyes:* anticholinergic effects (see above); retinitis pigmentosa with long-term thioridazine; risk of cataract described in dogs given high-dose quetiapine, but not seen in excess in humans at therapeutic dose
- *Sexual side effects:* common, and a potential cause of non-adherence, but often missed by the clinician; mechanisms complex and multifactorial but hyperprolactinaemia is a recognized association.

The usual strategy is for a slow tapering of the extant agent, with a cross-taper over days to weeks with the new agent. However, each switch needs to be customized to the individual, and should take into account the following:

1. The dose of agent switching from
2. The target dose of agent switching to

3. The side effect profile of each agent (e.g. switching from a sedating agent to a non-sedating agent can result in break-through insomnia)
4. The setting (e.g. inpatient switch can be more rapid as close clinical monitoring is available).

Common problems arising during the switch, and how to manage them, are outlined in Box 8.4.

8.4 **What are the particular precautions to be taken in administering clozapine?**

Because of clozapine's unique place in the pharmacological armamentarium, as well as its potentially fatal side effects, special care needs to be taken in its use. A full review of the patient's medical and treatment history needs to be obtained, to ensure they have had satisfactory trials of at least two antipsychotics from different classes of antipsychotic agent. Some clinicians consider that the trial of a typical agent is warranted before clozapine, but others prefer to use clozapine earlier in the treatment algorithm. The patient and (where feasible) their family should be involved in a detailed discussion about the rationale and potential risks and benefits of clozapine. A handout such as that provided in the Appendix of this book can be provided, and other resources such as videos are available from the manufacturers.

The patient is usually admitted to hospital to commence clozapine, and a slow dose titration is required, with 12.5mg on day 1, increasing by 25–50mg per day over the first 10 days. The optimal dose is dependent upon clinical response and side effect profile, but usually the effective dose is in the range 200–450mg per day. Blood levels can also be helpful to guide dosing: levels of > 600ng/mL are associated with higher rates of symptom control.

Details of blood testing and other monitoring are shown in Figure 8.2, which also provides a monitoring template. *Haematological tests* must be performed and results checked prior to prescribing the agent: the interval is usually weekly for the first 18 weeks, and monthly thereafter. Certain pre-defined cut-off points for total white cell and

---

Box 8.4 Problems arising during switching of antipsychotics, and how to counter them

- *Cholinergic rebound*: short-term anticholinergic agent
- *Rebound psychosis or EPSE*: slow cross-titration; symptomatic treatment with benzodiazepine
- *Rebound insomnia*: short-term hypnotic agent.

Figure 8.2 Clozapine monitoring

ST VINCENT'S
MENTAL HEALTH
CLOZAPINE MONITORING

INSTRUCTIONS FOR USE:
- Complete for the first 18 weeks and then use Metabolic Monitoring Form on an ongoing basis.
- An authorised signed entry to be completed in the medical record/progress notes for each measure on each occasion.
- Filing: this form should be filed in the Mental Health forms section of the record in order of most recent date of entry.

UR No.: _____
Surname: _____
Given Name: _____
D.O.B.: _____
Please fill in if no Patient Label available

Clozapine Patient No. (CPN): _____

Patient Height: ____ (m)   RAPID No: _____

		BASE	1	2	3	4	5	6	7	8	9	10	11	12	13	14	15	16	17	18
	Base Date / /																			

(Insert Date of Procedure in unshaded cells)

Week

Key Investigations
- FBE – Taken in the last 7 days / Monthly after 18 weeks WCC Neutrophil Eosinophil
- Blood Group
- BHCG (Females where appropriate)
- LFTs
- U&Es
- Troponin I/CK

Metabolic Syndrome X
- Fasting Blood Glucose
- Blood Pressure
- Lipids (Chol, LDL, HDL, TG)
- Weight (Kg)
- BMI = weight in kg by height or m²
- Waist Measurement (cm)

Cardiac
- Echocardiogram (pre-commencement and 6 weeks)
- ECG

Physical
- Temperature
- Pulse
- Respiratory Rate

Serum Clozapine

ST VINCENT'S MENTAL HEALTH – CLOZAPINE INITIATION

SV 655 07/07

CHAPTER 8 **Pharmacological & physical**

71

> **Box 8.5 White blood count (WBC) and neutrophil count (NC) cut-offs with clozapine**
>
> • *Green*: WBC > 3.5 and NC > 2.0: continue to prescribe, and continue weekly or monthly blood tests, dependent upon stage of treatment.
> • *Amber*: WBC 3.0–3.5 and/or NC 1.5–2.0: continue to prescribe, but perform blood tests twice weekly till normalizes.
> • *Red*: WBC < 3.0 and/or NC < 1.5: STOP clozapine immediately; discuss with haematologist regarding best action; continue monitoring as advised by haematologist.

neutrophil counts (NC) require certain actions, as shown in Box 8.5. If a patient has had to have the drug withdrawn because of neutropaenia, any re-challenge needs to be performed in a very careful and controlled manner. Removing other agents that might suppress neutrophils (e.g. sodium valproate) is sensible if justifiable in terms of mental state. Some clinicians add low-dose lithium to enhance neutrophil production.

Cardiac monitoring is somewhat variable across centres. Certainly monitoring of pulse and blood pressure during the initial days of treatment should be routine. The use of troponin assays can be useful in detecting myocarditis. Routine echocardiograms (baseline, at 6 weeks, and then annually) have been adopted in some centres, though the exact 'yield' from such investigations is not clear.

Sedation can be a problem for some patients, and timing of the dose at a particular time in the evening should be tailored to the individual to try to minimize impact on daily activities. *Sialorrhoea* can also be both distressing and stigmatizing. Using a towel over the pillow at night, and/or atropine drops on the tongue can be helpful. *Enuresis* is also fairly common, presumably due to a combination of anticholinergic and sedative effects. Avoidance of fluids close to bedtime and emptying the bladder before retiring at night can avert this problem. *Myoclonic jerks and epileptiform seizures* are particularly common with clozapine use, and the effect is dose dependent. Addition of an anticonvulsant may be required. Sodium valproate is often used but carries the risk of increased weight gain in conjunction with clozapine. Carbamazepine should be avoided as it can suppress bone marrow.

As outlined earlier, clozapine also carries a high risk of weight gain, and is associated with emergent diabetes and hyperlipidaemia. Thus, routine tests for the metabolic syndrome are important, as they are for the other antipsychotics (see Section 8.2 and Figure 8.1).

8.5 Are combinations of antipsychotics ever justified?

The use of more than one antipsychotic agent at the same time has a very limited evidence base, and pharmacological purists eschew the practice. However, in patients who have residual symptoms in certain domains, or who experience particular side effects but a good clinical response to a particular agent, the use of combinations has clinical appeal. For example, studies have shown that adding quetiapine to clozapine can allow a reduction in the clozapine dose, with subsequent weight reduction; aripiprazole and ziprasidone are also being used by clinicians to counter weight gain and alleviate sedative side effects associated with other antipsychotics. These practices are mostly pragmatic, and carry the risk of drug–drug interactions and worsening of other side effects.

An area where combinations are probably sometimes justified is in people who simply do not respond optimally to any single agent, and in whom a combination is effective and well tolerated. Having said this, the preferred approach would be of optimal dosing of a series of single agents for a reasonable period (6–12 weeks) before resorting to combinations.

Suboptimal response to clozapine leaves the clinician with limited options, and adjunctive use of relatively 'clean' dopamine-D2 receptor antagonists (notably risperidone and amisulpride) has currency in clinical practice. The evidence for the use of adjunctive risperidone is equivocal at best, and there is very little well-researched data on amisulpride augmentation. Having said this, many clinicians have seen benefits from these combinations at an individual patient level. One of the plusses is that any EPSE-inducing properties of the adjunctive agent are usually reduced by the inherent properties of clozapine, including its strong antimuscarinic effects.

8.6 What adjunctive pharmacological treatments might be useful?

It is very common in clinical practice for people with schizophrenia to be prescribed more than one psychiatric medication. Adjunctive use of mood-stabilizing anticonvulsants or lithium is particularly popular. Certainly in patients with a strong affective flavouring to their illness, this has strong appeal, though again side effects of the combinations can be problematic (e.g. weight gain). Valproate also appears to have efficacy against aggressive behaviours, and has been shown to 'bring forward' antipsychotic response in the acute phase of treatment. Lamotrigine is favoured as an adjunct in many European countries, and there is emerging research evidence to support this practice; care needs to be taken to titrate the agent up slowly, to reduce the risk of adverse skin problems. Topiramate is used in some centres, but more for its weight loss propensity than as a mood stabilizer. Lithium has a place in the treatment of schizoaffective disorder, but needs to be taken regularly and the usual monitoring systems need to be in place (see Figure 8.1).

Other combinations are usually guided by the presence of 'comorbid' psychiatric conditions. Antidepressants, for example, are an important part of the treatment of depressive and anxiety symptoms, as detailed in Chapter 3. Again, drug–drug interactions need to be borne in mind; for example, fluvoxamine can cause massive rises in clozapine levels. Other agents used to treat anxiety in schizophrenia include buspirone and benzodiazepines; the latter, of course, carry a risk of dependence and need to be closely monitored.

8.7 **Are there effective treatments for negative symptoms?**

Negative symptoms, along with cognitive dysfunction, are strongly associated with disability in schizophrenia. It is thus concerning that our ability to treat negative symptoms is still very limited. As outlined earlier, the fact that at least the atypical antipsychotics tend not to make negative symptoms worse (as the typicals can) is a bonus. Also, most of the atypicals claim to be associated with some reduction in negative symptoms, though it can be difficult to know whether the effect is direct or via alleviation of positive symptoms, improved mood, or reduced EPSE which can result in 'secondary' negative symptoms (see Chapter 2).

The antipsychotics that have been best investigated for their action on primary negative symptoms are clozapine and amisulpride. Clozapine undoubtedly has an edge over other agents in treatment-resistant patients, including targeting negative symptoms. Amisulpride, at doses of 100–300mg daily, has shown benefit in trials of patients with predominantly negative symptoms ('deficit syndrome').

Other experimental approaches to the management of negative symptoms include the adjunctive use glycine, D-cycloserine, mirtazapine, galantamine, and pergolide. The evidence base for such interventions is slight, and further research is required to establish their true place in the treatment of schizophrenia.

Some non-pharmacological techniques have also been applied, with some success, to people with prominent negative symptoms. These include social skills training and cognitive behaviour therapy (CBT). These can be packaged to provide a comprehensive rehabilitation programme, including activity scheduling, graded tasks, environmental manipulation, and group-based social interaction sessions. It is also useful to include family members, at least to educate them about the nature of negative symptoms and thus reduce potential frustration and blaming (e.g. labelling the lack of motivation as simply 'laziness'). Families can also assist in expanding the individual's social repertoire.

8.8 Can we ameliorate cognitive dysfunction in schizophrenia?

As discussed earlier, some prescribed agents (such as anticholinergics) can make cognitive functioning worse, so these should be used very judiciously in clinical practice. Whether the newer 'atypical' antipsychotics enhance cognitive functioning is equivocal, though certainly they do not seem to make it worse, and some may have positive effects on certain domains of functioning. For example, clozapine appears particularly helpful in terms of amelioration of verbal fluency deficits and attentional problems, whilst aripiprazole has shown a fairly specific benefit for verbal learning. Other agents have been studied as potential cognitive enhancers. These include amphetamine-like agents (but these carry the risk of exacerbating psychotic symptoms) and nicotinic agonists.

Apart from pharmacological means, psychologists and others have investigated whether exercising the brain can enhance cognition. In this 'cognitive enhancement therapy', participants are given repeated paper-and-pencil and computer-based tasks of increasing complexity, repeated over and over. They certainly can show improvement in terms of those specific tasks, but how far these improvements generalize to other cognitive domains is not clear. Of considerable practical importance, however, is the fact that cognitive enhancement therapy, when integrated into a supported employment programme, can markedly improve work participation rates. As vocational enhancement is a major deficit in our treatment of people with schizophrenia, this research is very encouraging; we wait to see how widely it can be adopted beyond research and specialist settings.

8.9 What are the future directions for the biological treatment of schizophrenia?

It is somewhat ironic that our modern antipsychotics are no better at the alleviation of positive symptoms than were such original agents from the 1950s. It is also chastening that clozapine remains, after nearly 40 years, our most powerful and broadly effective antipsychotic. Also, despite some furious attempts to discredit or supplant it, the dopamine hypothesis is still arguably the best all-encompassing explanatory model for schizophrenia at a chemical level. But advances have been made, and certainly our newer antipsychotics are less burdensome in terms of key side effects such as EPSE and TD. Our understanding of serotonergic effects and glutamatergic influences on the pathophysiology of schizophrenia have brought, and continue to promise, more sophisticated treatments for the condition. Other systems, such as the muscarinic anticholinergic system, also hold potential promise in this regard. The holy grail for pharmacological treatments, though, remains negative and cognitive symptoms, which are at once so damaging and so elusive. Specific treatment approaches, such as medications targeting glutamatergic and nicotinic systems, hold some promise here. The cannabinoid system remains relatively under-explored in the treatment of schizophrenia, and warrants more investigation.

We also hold out hope that genetic investigations may lead us to a better understanding of the biology of schizophrenia, and thereupon to targeted drug development. There is also a good chance that pharmacogenomic advances will enable better prediction of an individual's chances of responding to (or getting certain side effects from) a particular medication. Such advances, particularly as the rest of medicine looks forward to 'personalized medicine', could totally alter the playing field in treating schizophrenia. Similarly, if other neurobiological (e.g. brain imaging, neurochemical) studies reveal ways to predict treatment response and/or relapse, then our approaches to treating schizophrenia could be radically altered for the better. On reflection, the pace of psychopharmacological drug development might seem too slow for real ('breakthrough') discoveries that can relieve the disabilities associated with schizophrenia. Nevertheless, the potential of science to change treatment expectations fundamentally is immense; in our lifetime perhaps the best example is of the discovery of AIDS being followed quickly by disease-altering vaccines. Patients and their families should always remain (cautiously) optimistic that research will ultimately 'deliver the goods' for them.

8.10 Is there a role for ECT and TMS in treating schizophrenia?

Electroconvulsive therapy (ECT) was arguably the first 'biological' treatment for schizophrenia, and was widely used until the advent of the antipsychotic medications in the 1950s. The use of ECT in clinical practice is now largely confined to patients with severe intractable depression, but there is still a role in some people with schizophrenia, as shown in Box 8.6.

> ### Box 8.6 Potential uses of ECT in schizophrenia
> - Patients with catatonia
> - Patients with concomitant severe depression unresponsive to antidepressants
> - Patients with severe schizoaffective disorder
> - Patients who do not respond adequately to other interventions.

Transcranial magnetic stimulation (TMS) is a more modern technique involving the induction of an electric current through the use of magnetic fields. Most clinical trials in psychiatry have been in the area of depression, but a few studies have tried to assess efficacy for certain symptoms of schizophrenia. These include the following:

- Left dorsolateral prefrontal cortex stimulation to ameliorate negative symptoms
- Left temporoparietal cortex stimulation to reduce persistent auditory hallucinations.

Results of these studies have been mixed, and the precise role of TMS in schizophrenia is still to be determined.

Chapter 9

Psychological and psychosocial treatments

Key points
• Psychological therapies have a potential key role in the holistic management of the person with schizophrenia.
• Specific treatments targeting medication adherence, social anxiety, social skills, and illicit substance use have proven efficacy for people with schizophrenia.
• Promising results have been shown for treatments targeting medication-resistant delusions and hallucinations, though results have been somewhat inconsistent.
• Cognitive enhancement strategies have exciting potential in assisting people with schizophrenia to obtain and retain work.
• Overall, psychological and psychosocial treatments are not as broadly available as they should be, and remain a deficit in the care of many people with schizophrenia.

9.1 What is the role of psychological interventions for schizophrenia?

A multidisciplinary team approach is most helpful in aiding people with schizophrenia deal with their complex sets of problems across multiple domains. One particular group of interventions has an ever-expanding role in this regard, namely psychological therapies. For example, elements of cognitive-behaviour therapy (CBT) can be usefully applied to patients with schizophrenia, following the general principles outlined in Box 9.1.

- Psychoeducation
- Links between thoughts, actions, and emotions
- Utility of activities and structure in daily living
- Mapping of symptoms/mood/anxiety/stress
- Empowerment to deal better with symptoms
- Thinking traps and negative consequences of negative thinking.

More specialized psychological interventions include the following:

a) *Helping people deal with 'medication-resistant' delusions and hallucination*: a CBT framework is the most well-researched approach, and has proved successful, especially for delusions. This work can be done individually or in a group-based manner, and in the latter format participants can learn much from each other about strategies to help deal more effectively with ongoing psychotic symptoms, reduce the distress they cause, and stop them from dominating their lives.

b) *Cognitive remediation* using either pencil-and-paper or computer-based paradigms. As discussed below, these strategies can enhance workplace participation and job retention.

c) *Acceptance-commitment therapy*, which has also been trialed in people with schizophrenia, with promising initial results.

9.2 **Can we help people with schizophrenia socialize?**

There are a number of reasons behind social isolation in schizophrenia, as detailed in Box 9.2.

It is important to understand individual barriers to socialization, so that relevant interventions can be offered. For example, clinicians often assume that failure to socialize is consequent upon negative symptoms, whilst, in fact, many patients report a desire to socialize but are impeded by anxiety. There are effective interventions for social anxiety disorder (SAD) in association with schizophrenia, using CBT techniques with or without serotonergic antidepressants. An outline of a group-based CBT programme for SAD in schizophrenia is shown in Box 9.3.

Another well-established intervention for social impairment in schizophrenia is social skills training. Here the individual is instructed minutely regarding how to socialize, by breaking tasks into small steps: for example, what to say when meeting a stranger, how to shake

> **Box 9.2 Reasons for social impairment in schizophrenia**
>
> - Positive symptoms, notably persecutory delusions
> - Negative symptoms
> - Disorganization symptoms
> - Cognitive deficits
> - Depression
> - Anxiety
> - Lack of opportunity.

> **Box 9.3 Elements of a group-based CBT intervention for SAD in schizophrenia (from Halperin et al. 2000; Kingsep et al. 2003)**
>
> - *Session 1:* overview of anxiety and social anxiety; group reflection on own experiences and concerns regarding socialization; modelling of social behaviours and interactions if appropriate; setting homework exercises (behavioural tasks and capturing negative thoughts)
> - *Session 2:* review of past week, and of homework progress and barriers; more explicit overview of negative automatic thoughts and effect on mood and anxiety levels
> - *Session 3:* exposure exercise with role play and review of cognitive restructuring
> - *Session 4:* educational video of social phobia; further homework tasks
> - *Sessions 5–7:* repeated education, role play, homework, and reviews of achievements and barriers; sharing of learnt strategies amongst group members
> - *Session 8:* social outing; tips to ensure maintenance of gains; setting of future tasks and problem-solving how to deal with potential future setbacks.

hands, and how to keep appropriate eye contact. Whilst successful in teaching certain social skills, there are questions about how generalizable these skills are to a broader spectrum of social situations.

Lack of opportunity to socialize is a major barrier for many people with schizophrenia. Engagement with local drop in centres, attending outings and group activities, and support, encouragement and modelling by case managers can be very helpful.

9.3 **Can we enhance adherence to treatment?**

Medication adherence is a key part of preventing relapse. Indeed, Robinson and colleagues showed in their first episode sample that patients who did not take their medications were five times more likely to relapse over the ensuing 2 years.

Certain factors are associated with poor medication adherence, as shown in Box 9.4. It should be stressed, though, that non-adherence is a very individual business, and every attempt should be made to understand individual reasons for not taking medications, since successfully addressing these issues is the key to enhancing adherence in the longer term.

A number of approaches can be engaged to try to enhance adherence, as shown in Box 9.5.

Box 9.4 Associations of poor adherence to treatment in schizophrenia

Illness and sociocultural issues
- Lack of insight into the illness and the need for treatment
- Cognitive impairment
- Cultural beliefs against medication
- Lack of family support for treatment.

Medication issues
- Lack of a good therapeutic alliance
- Complex medication regimes
- Side effects of medication
- Perceived stigma associated with medication.

Box 9.5 Examples of adherence enhancement strategies

- Psychoeducation, including about medication and side effects
- Empowering patient to take responsibility for staying well
- Use of normalizing techniques (e.g. other chronic illnesses such as diabetes or hypertension)
- Explication of pros and cons of medication
- Dealing effectively with side effects
- Linking medication to routine everyday activity (e.g. brushing teeth)
- Monitoring adherence, using diary or calendar
- Blister packs or dosette boxes
- Long-acting injectable forms.

One powerful tool in the quest for enhanced medication adherence is the use of long-acting injectable forms of antipsychotics. Until recently, only the older typical agents such as zuclopenthixol, fluphenazine, flupenthixol, and haloperidol were available in long-acting injectable form. These are constituted in an oily base and are given as a deep intramuscular injection at intervals of anything from 2 to 4 weeks. The major down side of these agents is that they carry the burden of extrapyramidal side effects (EPSEs) associated with their parent compounds (see Section 8.2). Thus, the advent of a long-acting form of the atypical agent risperidone has been most welcome. Risperidone, long-acting (Risperdal Consta®), is constituted as an aqueous solution with the active agent in 'microspheres' of glycolic acid. It is given at fortnightly intervals at doses from 25mg to 50mg; some patients show added benefit with few side effects at doses up to 100mg every 2 weeks. As it takes some weeks to reach steady state, cover with oral risperidone is required over the first 5 to 6 weeks. A long-acting form of olanzapine (Relprev®) is also now available. It is embedded in a palmoate salt and is given once a month. A long-acting form of another drug—paliperidone—that has a monthly administration regimen is also currently under regulatory review.

9.4 How do we deal with physical health risks associated with schizophrenia?

As outlined in Part 1 of this book, people with schizophrenia carry a high burden of physical health problems, and tragically such problems are often unrecognized and are certainly often under-treated. Thus, optimal monitoring and appropriate interventions should be mandated in clinical practice. Given that the medications psychiatrists prescribe can exacerbate a number of these physical health issues, it would seem appropriate for that group to take a lead in this endeavour.

Various monitoring systems have been developed to assist clinicians and services to monitor physical health parameters over extended periods. An example is shown in Figure 8.1. It is important that the patient is a partner in this process, and they can be encouraged to carry their own copy of the monitoring form, ensuring that tests are performed at the required times and that they understand the results of such tests. The patient's general practitioner can usefully be incorporated into the monitoring system, ensuring that tests are interpreted correctly and appropriate interventions are followed.

Healthy lifestyle packages have been developed and tested by a number of researchers, and incorporated into clinical practice in many settings. Elements usually encompass regular monitoring and inclusion of the patient in this process, psychoeducation, promotion of healthy eating (involvement of a nutritionist can be most helpful), and exercise regimes. Barriers include motivating the patient, enabling participation in gyms, and ensuring that the regime continues over the long term (gains are quickly lost if not consistently adhered to). Group work has the potential benefit of cost-effectiveness of delivery and the camaraderie, support, and encouragement of fellow group members. Medications that have shown some promise in weight reduction in some people with schizophrenia include sibutramine, orlistat, topiramate, and nizatidine. Cannabinoid CB1 receptor antagonists such as rimonabant may also have a role to play, though depression is a potentially worrying side effect. With any pharmacological intervention, caution needs to be shown in monitoring interactions and side effects.

Cigarette smoking requires particular emphasis, and all too often clinicians simply accept that 'everyone with schizophrenia smokes'. Education about the adverse health risks of smoking is imperative, and arrangement with local 'quit' agencies should be fostered. Nicotine replacement programmes, in conjunction with cognitive-behavioural packages, have proved effective in schizophrenia patients, and bupropion can be safely used unless there are drug–drug interactions. Newer agents worthy of investigation in this group include rimonabant and varenicline, though both carry a risk of mood disturbance and so need careful monitoring.

9.5 How can we assist patients who abuse alcohol and illicit substances?

There is little doubt that alcohol and illicit substance use are major problems for many people with schizophrenia. Rates of use are markedly elevated, notably of illicit substances, and the use of such agents has adverse consequences for the longitudinal course of illness, as outlined earlier. Furthermore, the major consensus finding from the literature, namely that both sets of problems should be dealt with in an integrated manner, is often not delivered on, by clinicians. It is particularly worrisome that services are often not configured well to deal with both mental health and substance use problems simultaneously. Many people with these dual problems are left to 'fall between the cracks', and neither set of issues is adequately dealt with.

Solutions are not easy to come by, because service reconfiguration is often bedevilled by vested interests and 'historical' practice. But the fact that over 60% of people with a mental health problem have a substance use disorder (SUD), and a similar proportion of SUD service users have a mental illness, speaks to the necessity for clinicians in both types of service to be cognizant of these risks, to screen for them routinely, and either deliver or refer for appropriate treatment of each problem. It is also critical that effective communication occurs between SUD and mental health services, such that clear and consistent messages are given to the patient.

Mental health workers should, in particular, ensure they screen for SUD in their patients and are comfortable with motivational interviewing techniques, which can assist getting 'pre-contemplative' patients to start looking more concertedly at their SUD as a problem. Useful questions to ask the pre-contemplative patient include 'What sort of thing could occur to make you start thinking that your substance use might be a problem for you?'; and 'How will you know when it is time to quit?'. Also, working through a 'decisional balance' (weighing pros and cons) with respect to substance use can help the individual see their substance use in a more objective way. Mapping substance use and mental health problems on a single matrix allows clinician and patient to understand patterns, recognize high-risk situations, and establish interactions between the two sets of problems.

The problem of medication adherence is particularly challenging in this patient group. They do not take their prescribed medications because they do not work well enough or they dislike their side effects. This patient group has, particularly, low tolerance for side effects, especially those like akathisia or even antipsychotic-induced negative symptoms which 'drive them to drink'. Also, the alcohol or drugs that they take will calm anxiety and reduce hallucinations—effects that doctors often fail to acknowledge even though patients know this well from their experiences. Of course, they worsen psychosis in the long run and compete with patient's efforts to maintain adherence with their prescribed medications. Education on the actual effects of drug and alcohol use is, therefore, an important component of care for these (and indeed for all) patients.

There are good examples of programmes that employ the effective components of both SUD and mental health, and that can be delivered by clinicians in either setting. These can be delivered individually or in a group-based manner, and have demonstrable benefits for both mental health and SUD, as well as more broadly for reduced service utilization, notably hospitalizations. An example of the elements of this programme is shown in Box 9.6.

> **Box 9.6 Elements of an integrated programme for mental health and substance use disorder (James et al. 2004)**
>
> Module 1:
> - Introduction
> - Drug education
> - The relationship between mental health and drug use.
>
> Module 2:
> - Enhancing motivation
> - Reasons for changing drug use
> - Goal setting.
>
> Module 3:
> - Ways to change
> - Harm reduction
> - Tips for cutting down
> - Self-monitoring.
>
> Module 4:
> - Coping in high risk situations.
>
> Module 5:
> - Review of sessions
> - Planning for the future
> - Meeting with case managers.

9.6 How can we help people with schizophrenia get into the workforce?

As outlined in Chapter 4, there are major barriers preventing the majority of people with schizophrenia gaining paid employment. To assist them, we need to work at both an individual level and a workplace level.

Interventions at the individual level: Supported employment programmes have been shown to benefit people with a mental illness. As part of this process, people with schizophrenia require direct assistance to attain and retain paid work (i.e. merely offering counselling or job interview training is inadequate); and vocational and clinical services need to be integrated rather than offered separately. Novel approaches to augmenting the benefits of supported employment are shown in Box 9.7.

> ### Box 9.7 Strategies to augment supported employment
>
> - *Behaviour feedback groups with goal setting:* workers meet on a regular basis with a facilitator to feed back to each other on work performance and other work-related issues, and set goals such as being more punctual or taking fewer breaks. This process enhances social skills and cooperativeness on the job, and provides a social learning opportunity.
> - *Cognitive behavioural interventions:* these challenge negative assumptions about work and work capacity and set behavioural goals.
> - *Social skills:* teaching of skill sets pertinent to the workplace, balancing the 'gives' and 'gets' related to work, and helping the individual identify and effectively negotiate potential problems.
> - *Cognitive enhancement:* computerized packages offered as an adjunct to other work support programmes improve workplace participation rates.

Workplace-level interventions: An alternative, though not mutually exclusive, approach is to address workplace issues themselves. At a general level, this entails educating potential employers about the nature of schizophrenia, and giving practical tips about how to support and effectively help work colleagues who might be exhibiting symptoms of the illness. Specific tips should be taught to supervisors, including the following:

- How to address mental health issues in a sensitive manner
- How to provide workplace flexibility (e.g. in terms of hours of attendance)
- Environmental issues
- Being prepared if things go awry and
- Accessing appropriate help when needed.

More focussed is the creation of workplaces specifically aimed at inclusion of people with a mental illness. These 'social firms' are commercial businesses with a social goal, and which have a workforce that includes usually around 25–50% people with a mental illness. They aim to provide accessible and supportive workplaces for people with illnesses such as schizophrenia, and can also provide vocational training opportunities.

9.7 How should we involve the family?

The importance of family environment for someone with schizophrenia has been alluded to in Part 1 of this book. All too often, families themselves feel stigmatized and alienated and at the very least need education and support. Referral to local support organizations can be very helpful, since families realize that they are not alone, and can learn useful strategies for helping themselves and their loved ones, and dealing with societal stigma.

Elements of effective family interventions in schizophrenia are shown in Box 9.8. In terms of specific family interventions, studies in many different countries and cultural settings have shown benefits for reducing expressed emotion in 'high EE' families; there are subsequent gains in terms of reduction in relapse and hospitalization.

Box 9.8 Elements of effective family interventions for schizophrenia

- Psychoeducation regarding the illness, its symptoms, its treatment, and side effects of medication
- Acknowledging and dealing with stigma, both within the family and within the wider community
- Problem-solving techniques for the family to attempt and refine
- Enhancement of communication between family members
- Addressing emotional issues and responses to the ill family member (e.g. blame, guilt)
- Encouraging extension of social networks and avoiding isolation of the family from broader society
- Ensuring the family's expectations of the ill family member are realistic
- Providing hope and encouragement.

Chapter 10

Special clinical situations

Key points
• Women with schizophrenia have a number of unique problems associated with the illness: these need to be acknowledged and addressed in a consistent manner.
• Early intervention in schizophrenia has the ability to 'get it right' from the beginning with respect to the patient and their family, and potentially help avoid later pitfalls.
• Treatment resistance is an ill-defined concept, and our ability to effectively help people who do not respond adequately to first- or second-line treatments remains limited.
• The management of the acutely unwell and potentially violent patient requires excellent clinical care, sensible pharmacotherapy, and measures to ensure that the dignity of the individual is not adversely affected.

10.1 Women with schizophrenia

Women with schizophrenia have a number of important particular issues to deal with as part of their illness process. Not least amongst these are issues relating to fertility and potential parenthood. Many women with schizophrenia desire children, and many have them, though regrettably they are all too often unplanned, with suboptimal antenatal care, poor nutrition, and high rates of cigarette smoking during pregnancy, adding to overall high rates of reproductive pathology. Added to this is the major hormonal flux that occurs after birth, and the stress of having a baby in an often unsupported domestic environment. Also, the pervasive fear that social services might remove the child results in many women in this scenario not seeking or receiving appropriate postnatal care. There is a major challenge for services to work closely together to ensure better care for women with schizophrenia.

Another issue is the use of medications during pregnancy and breast-feeding. Decision making here requires full discussion with the patient and (whenever feasible) her partner, of risks and benefits associated with either continuing or halting medication. Any potential harm to the developing foetus needs to be weighed against the very real risk of relapse should medication be discontinued.

Other problems for women with schizophrenia include the fact that oestrogen flux during menstrual cycles appears to impact psychotic symptoms, and antipsychotic medications can perturb menstrual regularity and cause sexual dysfunction. Furthermore, most psychotropic medications are tested on predominantly male patients, leaving deficits in our knowledge about side effects and appropriate doses in women: it is clear that pre-menopausal women require lower doses of antipsychotics than men, but all too often receive doses higher than is optimal for them.

10.2 What is so special about the first episode?

Many clinicians consider the first presentation of psychosis as a unique 'window of opportunity' in care to get it right from the beginning. Unfortunately, many patients may have been ill for a long time before they come to care. Some researchers contend that this period of florid psychosis in the absence of treatment—the so-called duration of untreated psychosis or DUP—makes the illness worse in the long run. Accordingly, several centres have begun public health campaigns to encourage people to recognize and seek help for early psychotic symptoms.

Another important aspect about first episode psychosis (FEP) is that it can be challenging to diagnose (in truth, the best diagnosis is made later on when you have had the chance to evaluate the patient over time). Patients can present with depressive symptoms, which can mimic (especially negative) symptoms of schizophrenia. They can—and often do—present with substance abuse problems. Here, the clinician is again faced with the 'chicken and egg' dilemma of teasing out whether the psychosis came first or whether the drug abuse brought on the psychosis. Guidance regarding this clinical dilemma is provided in Chapter 3, but often it is simply impossible to tell. In such circumstances, being clinically cautious is a sensible strategy, such that the patient and his/her family are not erroneously told that the diagnosis is schizophrenia—a potentially life-long affliction—when it might be a drug-induced psychosis. Conversely, sometimes parents later on opine that their son/daughter with schizophrenia was told at their first psychotic episode that it was (simply) due to drugs. In this circumstance, parents often continue to be suspicious and distressed that an initial misattribution of diagnosis to drug abuse and the care thereupon could have contributed to the later chronicity of the their loved one's illness.

So, diagnostic skills are really important in FEP. Also, how and what explanation is given to the patient and their family really matters, both immediately and in the longer term. People mostly tolerate genuine uncertainty on the part of the clinician better than a forth-right proclamation of a definitive diagnosis. Often, they are even relieved if the clinician gives a 'working diagnosis' with assurance that it will be revisited later.

Finally, it is prudent to check for potential medical causes of an acute psychosis. It is likely that all investigations (physical examina-tion, blood tests, and a brain scan) will turn out to be normal. Nevertheless, even if the patient does have schizophrenia, the patient and their family will value the assurance that a proper diagnostic evaluation was performed at the beginning of the illness, and 'reversi-ble' organic causes excluded. Indeed, this is an important aspect in helping families to come to terms with the diagnosis of schizophrenia. This also helps to build their trust in the competence of this new doctor in their lives.

Regarding treatment options, it is appropriate to start an antipsy-chotic after informed consent. The informed consent process can be tricky because the patient and their family need to be fully informed about the rationale for the use of the medication, as well as potential risks such as weight gain and diabetes (see Chapter 3). At the same time, one does not wish to frighten them off at the first time when they learn about the illness and the available treatments.

There is no definitive guidance on which antipsychotic to choose to begin with, but reference to clinical tips such as those provided in Box 8.1 can be useful in tailoring the medication to the individual. Most patients respond well to medication, with a reduction of posi-tive symptoms particularly. But this can take weeks or even months (up to 37 weeks on average in one FEP study). Also, it is not clear when the medication is started, as to whether the patient will regain their pre-morbid level of functioning, or whether they will be left with residual impairment, or whether they will show a poor response to medications from the beginning. The earlier the onset of illness, the more insidious its presentation is, and the presence of negative symptoms are all pointers to a poorer long-term course of schizophrenia (see also Box 4.1). It is important to convey the message in a hopeful and positive (yet cautious) way to the patient and their family because most patients respond well to their initial treatment.

Generally, FEP patients require lower doses of antipsychotics than do patients with chronic schizophrenia. This is a good thing because it lessens the likely burden of side effects. This is particularly important because of the high likelihood that the patients will stop their medication if they experience side effects. Indeed, there is a high likelihood anyway that patients will try to go without medication at some stage after their psychotic symptoms have resolved. After all, one would not expect to take antibiotics indefinitely after a respiratory infection. As Dr Nina Schooler points out (personal communication, February 2008), this is often how patients and their families conceptualize the FEP and the role of medications. The clinician has to walk a fine line between conveying hope while still emphasizing the seriousness of the situation that requires long-term treatment. Also, it is not certain how long one should continue antipsychotic treatment. Some clinicians say for a year, some say for up to 3 or 5 years, and some say even indefinitely (a tough message to 'sell' at this early stage).

In addition to medication, the patient needs support from family and friends in an effort to 'hold on' to their life activities (e.g. studies or work) and not to lose their way at this vulnerable stage of their life. There is also the need (formal or informal) to express grief and to come to an understanding about what this new diagnosis could mean for the patient and his/her family. Stigma of mental illness might loom large. Depression might also set in. And so, for clinicians, it is important to devote lots of time to the support of both the patient and their family to work through their questions and concerns. Support groups, books, and the Internet are all helpful resources at this stage.

10.3 What can we do when patients prove 'resistant' to treatment?

Although the benefits of newer atypical antipsychotic medications are widely extolled, there remains a substantial minority of patients who do not respond adequately to antipsychotic therapy. There is also no real evidence that the proportion of patients who might be considered 'non-responders' has decreased to any large extent with second-generation antipsychotics. Moreover, despite the ongoing addition of new antipsychotics that the clinician can use in 'non-responder', 'treatment refractory', or 'hard-to-treat' patients (there is no clear term or uniform definition yet for 'treatment resistance'), clozapine remains 'the gold standard' for this group of patients. It is perhaps ironic then to observe that clozapine's use has essentially declined over time. Two important pragmatic trials mentioned in Chapter 8 (CATIE and CUtLASS) demonstrate that clozapine is more effective than other drugs for treatment refractory schizophrenia. So, when should a clinician decide that 'enough is enough' and that clozapine treatment is warranted? There is no consensus yet, but many would say that after two adequate trials ('adequate' means being long enough—probably 8 weeks—on the antipsychotic at an appropriate/high dose—nominally at least the equivalent of 300mg of chlorpromazine per day) of antipsychotic medications from different classes, clozapine should be considered next. Box 10.1 provides clinical guidance regarding this scenario.

If the patient is commenced on clozapine, it is important to monitor closely for both efficacy (getting plasma levels may help guide dosing of clozapine) and for side effects: for details of this process, the reader is referred to Chapter 8. the Appendix of this book contains a special section containing information for patients about to commence on clozapine, and Figure 8.2 provides a template for monitoring for potential side effects.

What to do next when clozapine does not work well enough is 'anyone's guess'. The options for augmentation strategies (either to treat general symptoms or to target negative or cognitive symptoms) have been described in Chapter 8. Suffice it to say that no one treatment stands out as a preferred option. There is ongoing research now to investigate whether the by-product of clozapine—N-desmethylclozapine—can deliver similar benefits as the parent compound, with a less burdensome adverse effect profile.

Obviously, in these patients all efforts must be made to support a reasonable and appropriate level of functioning, given the limitations of persistent psychotic symptoms. In this circumstance, Assertive Community Treatment (ACT) and other psychosocial supports (see Chapters 7 and 9) are key to optimizing functional performance.

Box 10.1 General management strategies for refractory schizophrenia

- Confirm prior treatment trials history and medication adherence.
- Evaluate for physical and psychiatric/substance abuse comorbidities.
- Consider high doses (with caution) of second-generation antipsychotic medication.
- Consider clozapine—evaluate and monitor accordingly.
- Clozapine augmentation strategies are unclear and largely unproven.
- Assertive Community Treatment (ACT) and other psychosocial supports are key to optimizing functional performance in persistently ill patients.

10.4 **How can we deal with acute behavioural disturbance in schizophrenia?**

It is essential to be ever vigilant for signs that a patient with schizophrenia is becoming agitated and/or more disturbed. Many of the features are the same as in somebody in the general public who get 'all worked up'—they pace, clench their fists or teeth, are loud and pressured in speech, and invade one's personal space. In addition, the patient might be preoccupied with internal stimuli (hearing things, seeing things) or may be directly threatening as a result of persecutory delusions or hearing voices commanding them to hurt someone. Alcohol or drug use may be another contributory factor, heightening the risk of violence through intoxication and disinhibition effects. Whatever the cause or circumstances, it is imperative to pick up the early warning signs and to intervene decisively and calmly, before things escalate. If possible, it is worth trying to move the patient to a quiet, safe room (remove all items that could be potential missiles). Get help—often a 'show of force' of several others present who are firm but not threatening or antagonistic can help the person regain control. Clearly, relatives and others who know the person well (e.g. a case manager) may be able to assist in calming the situation: however, care needs to be displayed in not exposing them to risk of being harmed, as it is clear that the patient's loved ones are the people who are most frequently the target and recipient of the patient's aggression.

Sometimes the patient will need to be physically restrained and/or placed in a seclusion ('quiet' or 'time-out') room. This is not a step to be taken lightly. Patients usually hate it and they may feel humiliated by the process. Obviously, it does little to help develop trust and a therapeutic relationship. Also, there have been far too many deaths of psychotic patients who were placed in seclusion and restraint. In the United States, many facilities have banned the use of these approaches, and seclusion-reduction strategies are in place in many other countries.

Frequently, agitation or actual aggression in a psychotic patient will be managed by giving some medication to 'calm them down'. It is an important principle in psychopharmacology that there is no drug actually approved directly to treat aggression (in contrast to analgesics which treat pain, or antipyretics to manage fever). Drugs that are often used in this situation include a fast-onset benzodiazepine (e.g. lorazepam), a first-generation antipsychotic, a second-generation antipsychotic (not clozapine), or a mood stabilizer (e.g. valproic acid). There is no compelling evidence that one drug is better than another in terms of calming, although several studies of second-generation antipsychotics point to these agents, perhaps, having more of a 'calming' than sedative effect and they are certainly less likely than the older agents to cause distressing and potentially dangerous extrapyramidal side effects (see Chapter 8).

Often, doctors have a particular drug or drug combination that they have both experience and confidence with. Algorithmic approaches (see reference list) have the advantage of guiding clinical practice, but should not be seen as prescriptive. It is, by patient choice, better to use a tablet, wafer, or liquid form of medication. However, it is often the case that by the time medications become a preferred management strategy, the patient is out of control and refuses to take medication voluntarily. In that instance, given the imminent risk of harm to self or others, medication can be given by acute-acting intramuscular injection. Whatever approach is taken, it is essential to monitor the patient carefully. Although, before being medicated the patient may have been at greater risk of harm to others, once medicated the risk shifts to them and the patient is liable to acute side effects. Akathisia can make agitation worse. Acute dystonia is very distressing and a therapeutic nightmare. Sedation and low blood pressure can be medically dangerous.

The patient needs to be carefully monitored in a safe and secure environment, expressly after the administration of parenteral medication. An opportunity should be provided for the patient (and if appropriate, the staff) to ventilate about their feelings, after such episodes.

Part 3

Appendix

Information for patients and carers

We have stressed throughout this book the importance of information for patients and carers about their illness and the treatments available to them. Many organisations and pharmaceutical companies have produced such information, and there is a plethora of websites offering advice and guidance. However, many clinicians prefer to be able to direct their patients to material which they themselves have seen, and which is clearly not linked to any particular pharmaceutical product. Thus, we reproduce here sections of a pamphlet developed at St Vincent's Hospital in Melbourne, Australia, by David Castle and Nga Tran (senior mental health pharmacist). It has been trialed with numerous consumers and carers and refined with their input. The full pamphlet covers all the main psychiatric medications, and is available from Professor Castle on david.castle @svhm.org.au.

Medication as part of the treatment of schizophrenia: information for patients and carers

Disclaimer

The information contained in this section is not intended to be a substitute for medical care. Decisions regarding treatment are complex medical decisions requiring the independent, informed decision of an appropriate healthcare professional. Reference to any drug or substance does not imply recommendation by the authors who accept no responsibility for any clinical untoward event that may arise from following the recommendations contained herein.

The role of medication in the treatment of schizophrenia

Most of us routinely take medicine for physical illnesses. If we have a cough or cold we use decongestants, throat lozenges and nasal spray. When we get a headache we take an aspirin without giving it a second thought. Many people don't realise that most mental and psychological illnesses often respond to medication. So, medication taken under a doctor's supervision, can play a valuable role in overcoming the symptoms of psychosis, and any associated mood and anxiety disorders. Medication may be a short-term therapy, or it may be required for a lengthy period. In some cases it may be required for many years, or even for life. In the treatment of the symptoms of schizophrenia, medications are used not just to help get you well, but also to keep you well. This is the same as for many physical illnesses such as diabetes, epilepsy and high blood pressure.

Finding the right medication

Many different drugs have proved useful in the treatment of mental disorders. Finding the right medication and dosage for each individual may require some detective work. Diagnosing the specific disorder will narrow the field of appropriate medication, and the doctor will make the final selection based on individual circumstances and your health history.

Each drug has advantages and disadvantages. Some work faster than others; some remain in the bloodstream longer. Some require several doses daily, others need to be taken only once a day. Medications' effectiveness varies with each individual. We are unique, and so is our response to medication. Sometimes the doctor will change dosages and switch medications to find the best match between the person and the medicine.

What the doctor should know

A doctor prescribing medication must know more about the person than just the illness being treated. A complete medical history is essential. To guard against counter productive or dangerous drug interactions, the doctor must know what other medications (including over-the-counter drugs, herbal remedies, other "natural products" or substances) you are taking or have taken recently. The doctor also needs to know about other medical problems or conditions that might affect treatment.

Risky combinations

Certain drugs should not be taken together. Some drugs can be dangerous when mixed with alcohol, particular foods, or other medications. You must be thorough and honest when the doctor asks about eating habits, health history and other drugs you are taking. Your own past experience with medication is also valuable information.

If you have been successfully treated with a specific drug in the past, that medication or one with similar properties might be preferable to an untried one. Likewise, the doctor would want to avoid prescribing a previously unsuccessful medication. Blood relatives often react to medication in a similar fashion, so experiences of family members can also be useful for the doctor to know.

Side effects and other reactions

Most people can take medications commonly used to treat mental and psychological disorders without difficulty, but sometimes there are side effects. Side effects vary with the drug but can range from minor annoyances like dry mouth or drowsiness to more troubling reactions like irregular heartbeat. **Fortunately, most side effects disappear in the first week or two of treatment. If the side effects persist, or if they interfere with normal activities, tell the doctor.** Potential side effects should be discussed before medication therapy begins. Knowing what to expect prevents unnecessary concern and alerts you to the kind of reactions that should be reported right away. Be sure to ask the doctor about side effects you might experience with your medication.

Scheduling and dosage

Getting the right result from medication depends on taking the right amount at the right time. Dosages and their frequency are determined by the need to ensure a consistent and steady amount of medication in the blood and by the length of time the drug remains active. If sticking to the schedule proves difficult, you should ask your doctor if adjustments can be made. Sometimes it is possible to change the timing of doses, although changes are not always possible.

You should not deviate from the prescribed dosages unless instructed by the doctor. People who have forgotten to take their medication at some point in the day are often tempted to "catch up" and take twice as much as prescribed at the next dose. Doubling up increases the risk of a bad reaction. The proper procedure is to take the right amount.

Believing that more is better, some people increase their dosage if their symptoms are not relieved immediately or because previous symptoms have returned. Others under-medicate themselves because they fear side effects. Some people cut back or stop medication on their own because their symptoms have disappeared. Cutting dosages or stopping medications can cause symptoms to return.

Special circumstances

Using medication is more complicated for some groups of people. Pregnant women and nursing mothers, for example, must avoid certain drugs because of possible danger to the infant. If you are pregnant or planning pregnancy, tell your doctor. Young children and the elderly also need special attention. Because of their lower body weight, youngsters generally are given smaller dosages of medication than adults. Treatment of the elderly may be complicated by co-existing health problems requiring other medications, which may not mix well with the new treatment.

Tips to help you take medication regularly

To help ensure you take your medication try to:

- Take it at a set time every day
- Link it to a regular activity such as brushing your teeth
- Keep a simple medication diary or mark it on a calendar when you take it
- Use a blister pack or dosette box from your pharmacy

How long will drug therapy last?

The length of drug therapy will vary with the individual and the severity of the disorder. You are likely to need medication for at least several months. Some people may need medication for a year or longer, even for life in some cases, to keep you well.

Medication therapy generally involves a regular dosage schedule but in cases of mild or infrequent anxiety or agitation you may be prescribed "PRN" medication to be taken at your discretion when needed. Stopping medication requires as much care as starting it. Medications should be phased out gradually under the direct supervision of your doctor.

Strategies to deal with common side-effects

- **Sedation** may be troublesome. Giving most of the dose at night may help, or a dose change may be required.
- **Weight Gain** can be a problem with some medications. Maintaining a healthy diet and getting plenty of exercise is recommended. Your doctor can assist you in obtaining dietary advice.
- **Dry Mouth**: try taking sips of water with a bit of lemon juice in it, lemon & glycerine swabs, sucking ice, sugarless gum etc. If none of these strategies work, ask your pharmacist about artificial saliva.
- **Constipation** can be a persistent problem. A diet high in fibre and drinking plenty of water and moderate exercise is recommended.
- **Light-headedness**, dizziness or giddiness on standing can be a problem particularly. If you get dizzy on standing, sit down, wait a little, then slowly get up again.
- **Nausea** can occur in the first weeks of treatment. An antinauseant medication may be needed.

Common medications in psychiatry

Psychiatric medications used are divided into several distinct groups based on their chemical properties. The following provides an overview.

Antipsychotics

Are used to treat many mental & psychological disorders such as schizophrenia, mania, psychotic depression and drug induced psychosis. Depending on the condition being treated, they may be required to be taken for a few months, or in some cases for several years. They take several weeks to work, and if they are stopped too soon the symptoms they are being used to treat will often return.

Antidepressants

SSRIs (Selective Serotonin Reuptake Inhibitors) and SNRIs (Serotonin Noradrenaline Reuptake Inhibitors) are now considered first-line treatment for depression. Their safety & convenience (they require once-a-day dosing) have made them among the most widely used drugs in the world. The most common side effects which tend to resolve after 3 or 4 weeks are mild nausea, headaches, restlessness and insomnia. Sexual dysfunction, primarily ejaculatory delay, also has been reported. They may cause sexual dysfunction in females too, particularly difficulty in attaining orgasm.

Noradrenaline and Specific Serotonin Antagonists (NaSSAs) and Noradrenaline Reuptake Inhibitors (NaRIs) are newer antidepressants with unique modes of action. The NaSSAs are associated with sedation and potentially weight gain, while the NaRIs are somewhat energising.

Tricyclic Antidepressants (TCAs) were among the first effective antide pressants but some are also effective for panic attacks and they may be used in the treatment of chronic pain syndromes. Tricyclics generally take two or three weeks to take effect. Side effects may include weight gain, drowsiness, dry mouth, dizziness and impaired sexual function.

Mood stabilizers

These are used to reduce the severity of mood swings and may also reduce irritability and aggression. All mood stabilizers require blood tests to monitor levels. Your doctor will also monitor blood, kidney function, thyroid & liver function where appropriate.

Lithium is a salt and may cause thirst, passing of large volumes of urine, and tremor. If dehydration occurs it may become toxic with harmful effects on the kidneys. Early warning signs of lithium toxicity may include nausea/vomiting, worsening tremor & severe drowsiness or confusion. If you have these symptoms and think you might be becoming lithium toxic you should go to your doctor or Emergency Department of the Hospital immediately.

Carbamazepine is an anticonvulsant, which also acts as an effective mood stabilizer. Side effects may include sedation, rash, double vision, dizziness and unsteadiness on the feet.

Sodium Valproate is an anticonvulsant which is also a very effective treatment for acute mania and is a mood stabilizer. Side effects can include nausea, weight gain, menstrual disturbance in females and tremor. Occasionally it can cause thinning of the hair.

Anxiolytics

Benzodiazepines are effective against anxiety and agitation. They are also used for the short term treatment of insomnia. Benzodiazepines are relatively fast-acting. Their principle side effect is drowsiness. They have the potential for dependency. There is often a temporary withdrawal syndrome when they are stopped suddenly. For these reasons benzodiazepines are usually only prescribed for a short period of time (less than 2 weeks).

Side effect medications

Anticholinergic drugs such as benztropine, benzhexol and biperiden are used to treat side effects of antipsychotic medications, mainly muscle stiffness or tremor. They may themselves cause side effects such as dry mouth, blurred vision and constipation. They should be prescribed with great care for those who suffer from glaucoma or have prostate problems as they can make these conditions worse.

Beta Blockers may also be used to reduce side effects from other medications, such as restlessness or tremor. They also reduce anxiety, reduce blood pressure and slow the heartbeat. They should not be taken by people who suffer from asthma.

Antipsychotic medications

What are antipsychotic medications for?

"Antipsychotics" are often effective in controlling psychotic symptoms and enable people to return to normal life. They are able to reduce or sometime alleviate the distressing and disabling symptoms such as hallucinations, disorganized thinking, altered perceptions of reality, mood swings, extreme fearfulness and severe agitation.

How do antipsychotic medications work?

Antipsychotic medications help to restore the brain's natural chemical balance, especially dopamine; hence, reducing or eliminating the psychotic symptoms. There are two groups of antipsychotic medications:

Atypical antipsychotics generally have fewer side effects than the older agents, especially extrapyramidal side effects such as rigidity, persistent muscle spasm, tremors, and restlessness. Also, they may be effective in improving mood, thinking and motivation.

Typical antipsychotics are older agents that are less popular nowadays because of the greater side effect burden described above.

Medications

Medication Class	Disorder for which Prescribed	Benefits	Drawbacks
Antipsychotics (typical) Chlorpromazine (Largactil®), Thioridazine (Aldazine®), Trifluoperazine (Stelazine®), Haloperidol (Serenace®, Haldol®), Flupenthixol (Fluanxol®), Zuclopenthixol (Clopixol®)	Psychosis, Schizophrenia, Schizo-affective Disorder Some also indicated for Bipolar Disorder	Effective for many people 2–4 weeks often needed for full response.	Side effects can include restlessness, tremor muscle stiffness constipation and weight gain.
Antipsychotics (atypical) Risperidone (Risperdal®), Olanzapine (Zyprexa®), Quetiapine (Seroquel®), Clozapine (Clopine®/Clozaril®), Amisulpride (Solian®), Aripiprazole (Abilify®), Sertindole (Serdolect®) Ziprasidone (Zeldox®)	Psychosis, Schizophrenia, Schizo-affective Disorder Some also indicated for Bipolar Disorder	Effective for many people 2–6 weeks often needed for full response. Clozapine reserved for 'treatment resistance'.	Most side effects much milder than with conventional drugs. Sedation and weight gain may be a problem with some agents.
Tricyclic Anti-depressants (TCAs), Imipramine (Tofranil®), Amitriptyline (Tryptanol®), Dothiepin (Prothiaden®), Doxepin (Sinepin®), Senequan®, Deptran®, Nortriptyline (Allegron®), Trimipramine (Surmontil®)	Depression Obsessive Compulsive Disorder (OCD) Panic Disorder Generalized Anxiety Disorder	Effective for many people; 2–4 weeks often needed for good response.	Dry mouth, constipation blurred vision dizziness, low blood pressure, moderate weight gain and occasionally difficulty in urinating.

Medication Class	Disorder for which Prescribed	Benefits	Drawbacks
Selective Serotonin Reuptake Inhibitors (SSRIs) Fluoxetine (Prozac®), Sertraline Zoloft®), Citalopram (Cipramil®), Paroxetine (Aropax®) Fluvoxamine (Luvox®), Escitalopram (Lexapro®)	Depression Obsessive Compulsive Disorder (OCD) Panic Disorder Generalized Anxiety Disorder	Effective for most people; once daily dosage. Often takes 2–4 weeks for response.	Nausea, insomnia, headache, nervousness; reports of delayed ejaculation.
Serotonin Noradrenaline Reuptake Inhibitors (SNRIs) Venlafaxine (Efexor® XL) Duloxetine (Cymbalta®) Desvenlafaxine (Pristiq®)	Major Depression Generalized Anxiety Disorder	Effective for many people; takes 2–4 weeks for response; will continue to improve after this.	Nausea, headache and insomnia may occur. Venlafaxine may raise blood pressure, especially at doses above 300mg/day.
Noradrenaline and Specific Serotonin Antagonist (NaSSA) Mirtazapine (Avanza® Mirtazon®, Axit®)	Major Depression Generalized Anxiety Disorder	Effective for many people; takes 2–4 weeks for response; will continue to improve after this.	Dry mouth, dizziness, sedation, weight gain.
Noradrenaline Reuptake Inhibitor (NARI) Reboxetine (Edronax®)	Major Depression	Effective for many people; takes 2–4 weeks for response; will continue to improve after this.	Urinary retention, dry mouth constipation, sweating, blood pressure increase, insomnia.

106

Medication Class	Disorder for which Prescribed	Benefits	Drawbacks
Mood Stabilzers Lithium (Lithicarb, Quilonum SR), Sodium Valproate (Epilim®), Carbamazepine (Tegretol®), Lamotrigine (Lamictal®), Topiramate (Topamax®)	Bipolar Disorder Depression (used to augment antidepressants) Sodium Valproate, Carbamazepine and Lamotrigine are also anticonvulsants.	Lithium may work within 1–2 days in some people, usually benefits seen with in 2 weeks. Valproate & Carbamazepine may work better than Lithium in 'rapid cycling' Bipolar Disorder. Lamotrigine is most effective for the depressed phase of Bipolar Disorder.	All mood stabilizers require regular blood monitoring. Lithium may cause side effects such a weight gain. Lamotrigine can cause serious skin problems and must be started slowly.
Benzodiazepines Lorazepam (Ativan®) Clonazepam (Rivotril®), Diazepam (Valium®), Alprazolam (Xanax®), Temazepam (Temaze®, Normison® Temtabs®), Nitrazepam (Mogadon®), Oxazepam (Serepax®)	Insomnia Anxiety Agitation	Fast acting with most people feeling better in the first week and many feeling the effects from the first day of treatment.	Habit forming; can cause drowsiness and interfere with concentration, driving and operating machinery.
Anticholinergics Benztropine (Benztrop®) Benzhexol (Artane®)	Side effects of antipsychotics such as muscle stiffness.	Enables side effects from antipsychotic medications to be managed.	Can cause dry mouth, blurred vision and constipation
Beta Blockers Propranolol (Inderal®, Deralin®)	Side effects such as anxiety restlessness, tremor	Enables side effects from antipsychotic medications to be managed.	Can lower blood pressure, may cause dizziness or fainting at first. Not to be taken by asthmatics.

Antipsychotics	
"Typical" Antipsychotics	"Atypical" Antipsychotics
Chlorpromazine (Largactil®)	Amisulpride (Solian®)
Flupenthixol (Fluanxol®)	Aripiprazole (Abilify®)
Fluphenazine (Modecate®)	Clozapine (Clozaril®, Clopine®)
Haloperidol (Serenace®, Haldol®)	Olanzapine (Zyprexa®)
Pericyazine (Neulactil®)	Quetiapine (Seroquel®)
Thioridazine (Aldazine®)	Paliperidone (Invega®)
Trifluoperazine (Stelazine®)	Risperidone (Risperdal®, Risperdal Consta®)
Zuclopenthixol (Clopixol®)	Sertindole (Serdolect®)
	Ziprasidone (Zeldox®)

How long will the antipsychotic medications take to work?

Antipsychotics begin to relieve agitation and sleep disturbances in about 1 week. Many people see substantial improvement by the fourth to sixth week of treatment. Since antipsychotics require time to work, **do not decrease or increase the dose or stop the antipsychotic without discussing with your doctor first**.

How long should you take this medication?

Following a first episode of psychosis, it is recommended that antipsychotic medication be continued for at least 1-2 years; this decreases the chance of becoming ill again. For individuals that have had a psychotic illness for several years or repeated psychotic episodes, antipsychotic medication should be continued indefinitely. This is similar to someone with diabetes requiring lifelong insulin.

What happens if a dose is missed?

Take it as soon as possible, as long as it is only a few hours after the usual time. Otherwise, wait until the next dose is due and take it as normal—do not try to catch up by doubling the dose.

Do they interact with other medications?

Antipsychotics can change the effect of other medications, or may be affected by other medication. Always check with your doctor or pharmacist before taking other drugs, vitamins, minerals, herbal supplements, and alcohol. **Always inform any doctor or dentist that you see that you are taking an antipsychotic medication**.

Do antipsychotics have any unpleasant side effects?

All medicines have side effects - even the ones you can buy without a prescription at a pharmacy, supermarket or health food store. The important things to remember are that not everyone will have the same unwanted side effects. Side effects usually occur early in the treatment, many of them will settle down after a few weeks, when the body has adapted to the medications.

Possible side effects of antipsychotic medications

Side Effect	Treatment
Muscle spasms, excessive rigidity, shaking, inner restlessness	These symptoms can be controlled with: Anticholinergic agents: benztropine, benzhexol. Beta blockers: propranolol. Benzodiazepines: diazepam, clonazepam, lorazepam
Drowsiness/Fatigue	This problem usually goes away with time. Use of other drugs that make you drowsy will worsen the problem. Avoid driving a car or operating machinery if drowsiness persists.
Dizziness	Get up from a lying or sitting position slowly; dangle your legs over the edge of the bed for a few minutes before getting up. If dizziness persists or if you feel faint, then contact your doctor.
Dry mouth	Sour candy, ice cubes, popsicles, and sugarless gum help increase saliva in your mouth; try to avoid sweet, calorie-laden beverages. Drink water and brush your teeth regularly.
Blurred Vision	This usually occurs at start of treatment and may last 1-2 weeks. Reading under a bright light or at a distance may help; a magnifying glass can be of temporary assistance. If the problem continues, discuss with your doctor.
Constipation	Increase bulk foods in your diet, drink plenty of fluids and exercise regularly. A bulk laxative or a stool softener helps regulate the bowels.
Weight Changes	Monitor your food intake. Maintaining a healthy diet and try to avoid foods with high fat content. Establish a regular exercise regime. Let your doctor know if you notice a rapid increase in your weight or waist measurement.
Nausea or Heartburn	If this happens, take the medication with food.
Change in Sexual Ability/Desire	Discuss with your doctor about other medications without this side effect and which may be an appropriate alternative for you.

General precautions

Avoid exposure to extreme heat and humidity since antipsychotics may affect your body's ability to regulate temperature changes and blood pressure.

Antipsychotics may increase the effects of alcohol, making you more sleepy, dizzy and lightheaded.

Antipsychotics can impair the mental and physical abilities required for driving a car or operating machinery. Avoid these activities if you feel drowsy or slowed down.

Do not break or crush the medication unless you have been advised to do so by your doctor or pharmacist.

Antacids interfere with absorption of these drugs in your stomach and therefore may decrease their effect. To avoid this, take the antacid at least 2 hours before or 1 hour after taking your antipsychotic.

Excessive use of caffeinated beverages (coffee, tea, colas, etc.) can cause anxiety, agitation and restlessness and counteract some of the beneficial effects of your medication.

Cigarette smoking can change the amount of antipsychotic that remains in your bloodstream; inform your doctor if you make any changes to your current smoking habit.

Do not stop antipsychotic medication suddenly as this may result in withdrawal symptoms such as nausea, dizziness, sweating, headache, sleeping problems, agitation and tremor, and also result in the return of psychotic symptoms.

Clozapine

What is clozapine?
Clozapine belongs to the group of medicines known as antipsychotics. This group of medicines is used mainly in the treatment of schizophrenia.

How does clozapine work?

Clozapine is used to control symptoms of schizophrenia such as hallucinations (hearing voices) and delusionary ideas. Clozapine is used in patients with schizophrenia for whom other antipsychotics have not worked or have caused severe side effects.

Things you must do while you are taking clozapine
You must have strict and regular blood tests while taking clozapine, due to the rare potential problems for your blood cells. **After starting on clozapine, you must have a blood test at least once a week for the first 18 weeks of treatment, thereafter at least every 4 weeks for as long as you are taking clozapine, and for one month after stopping the medicine**.

Why is it so important to keep taking clozapine?
When taken regularly, clozapine begins to relieve agitation within the first week. Many people see substantial improvement by the fourth to sixth week of treatment. **It is important to keep taking your clozapine even if you feel well as it is used not only to get you well, but also to keep you well**. This is similar to someone with diabetes requiring lifelong insulin.

What happens if I miss a dose?

Take it as soon as possible, as long as it is only a few hours after the usual time. Otherwise, wait until the next dose is due and take it as normal—do not try to catch up by doubling the dose.

If you have missed taking clozapine for more than two days, you must contact your doctor immediately—*do not start taking your regular clozapine dose again without consulting your doctor*.

What happens if I have taken too much?

Immediately contact your doctor or your local **Poisons Information Centre** for advice, or go to your local Emergency Department. Do this even if there are no signs of discomfort or poisoning. You may need urgent medical attention.

Interactions with other medication

Clozapine can change the effect of other medications, or may be affected by other medication. Always check with your doctor or pharmacist before taking other drugs, vitamins, minerals, herbal supplements and alcohol.

Cigarette smoking can also change the amount of clozapine that remains in your bloodstream; inform your doctor if you make any changes to your current smoking habit.

General precautions

- **CLOZAPINE SHOULD NOT BE STOPPED SUDDENLY**.
- **ALWAYS** consult the prescribing doctor or pharmacist about any concerns you have.
- Tell your doctor or pharmacist as soon as possible if you do not feel well while you are taking Clozapine.
- Clozapine may increase the effects of alcohol, making you more sleepy, dizzy and lightheaded.
- Clozapine can impair the mental and physical abilities required for driving a car or operating machinery. Avoid these activities if you feel drowsy or slowed down.
- Excessive use of caffeinated beverages (coffee, tea, colas, etc.) can cause anxiety, agitation and restlessness and counteract some of the beneficial effects of your medication.

Side effects
Common side effects of clozapine

Side Effect	Treatment
Tiredness and drowsiness (sedation) may be troublesome.	Giving most of the dose at night may help, or a dose change may be required. Contact your doctor if symptoms persist.
Weight gain	Monitor your food intake. Maintain a healthy diet and try to avoid foods with high fat content. Establish a regular exercise regime. Let your doctor know if you notice a rapid increase in your weight or waist measurement.
High temperature can occur in the first couple of weeks of treatment. Sore throat, mouth ulcers, any 'flu-like' symptoms such as swollen glands or other signs of infection	High temperature usually goes away. Nevertheless, contact your doctor to make sure there are not other causes, such as an infection, especially when the fever continues and you also have other symptoms too.
A fast heart beat even when you are resting is common in the first few weeks of treatment.	It usually goes away. Contact your doctor if it persists or if you experience chest pain or breathlessness at the same time.
Loss of bladder control, especially at night (bed wetting) can occur at any time during treatment	Changing the night dose of clozapine or limiting fluid intake before bedtime can be helpful. Contact your doctor if symptoms continue.
Dizziness, light-headedness or fainting on standing	Get up from a lying or sitting position slowly; dangle your legs over the edge of the bed for a few minutes before getting up. If dizziness persists or if you feel faint, then contact your doctor.
Increased saliva production may be bothersome at night	Contact your doctor, as there are medications that can reduce/overcome this problem.
Constipation can be a persistent problem	Increase bulk foods in your diet, drink plenty of fluids and exercise regularly. A bulk laxative or a stool softener helps regulate the bowels.
Nausea and vomiting can occur in the first week of treatment	If this happens, contact your doctor, as an anti-nauseant medication may be required.

Rare side effects of clozapine

Side Effect	Treatment
Agranulocytosis is a blood condition where the number of white blood cells may be reduced. This is important because these white blood cells are needed to fight infection.	There is no way of knowing who is at risk of developing agranulocytosis. However, with regular blood tests it can be detected early. If clozapine is stopped as soon as possible, the white blood cell numbers should return to normal.
Myocarditis is a condition where the heart muscle is inflamed or swelling.	If you develop a fast or irregular heartbeat that is present even when you are resting, together with rapid breathing, shortness of breath, chest pain, or dizziness or light-headedness, contact your doctor immediately or go to the Emergency Department at your nearest hospital. You may need to be referred to a cardiologist.
Seizures or fits can occur at any stage in treatment and are often related to the dose or dose-increase.	Contact your doctor immediately or go to the Emergency Department at your nearest hospital when seizures occur. Your clozapine dose may need to be reduced or you may need medication to control the seizures. Do NOT drive.
Diabetes, where blood sugar levels are high.	Contact your doctor immediately if you experience any signs of loss of blood sugar control such as excessive thirst, dry mouth and skin, flushing, loss of appetite, or voiding large amount urine.

Looking after your physical health

People with a mental illness are at increased risk for a number of medical conditions that can have a negative impact on quality of life and longevity. Also, some psychiatric medications have side effects that can increase the risk of certain medical conditions, notably heart disease. It is very important for people with a mental illness to be aware of these issues and to ensure their physical health is properly monitored and any problems appropriately treated.

Discuss these issues with your doctor and make sure you keep a record of your weight, waist measurement, and blood pressure.

We suggest you have certain blood tests done on a regular basis to monitor your physical health.

Suggested monitoring

Suggested monitoring (at least six monthly) will vary according to the individual, their particular risk factors, and their particular medications:

Measurement of:
- weight
- waist measurement
- blood pressure

Blood tests for:
- liver function
- kidney function
- fasting blood sugar (for diabetes)
- fasting blood fats ("lipid profile")

If you are on *lithium* you will need your thyroid hormone and lithium level measured every six months.

If you are on *sodium valproate* or *carbamazepine* you will need your blood count and blood levels done every six months.

If you are on *clozapine* you will need weekly blood tests for the 1st 18 weeks of treatment, and monthly thereafter; and tests of heart function (your doctor will arrange these for you).

Also, if you have any underlying heart problems or are on medication that might affect the heart (eg. ziprasidone, clozapine) you should have regular tests of your heart (an ECG).

References and further reading

Adams CE, Fenton M, David AS (2001). Systematic meta-review of depot antipsychotic drugs for people with schizophrenia. *British Journal of Psychiatry*, **179**: 290–9.

Addington D, Addington J, Schissel B (1990). A depression rating scale for schizophrenics. *Schizophrenia research*, **3**: 247–51.

Allen MH (2001). Managing the agitated psychotic patient: a reappraisal of the evidence. *Journal of Clinical Psychiatry*, **61**: 11–20.

Allison DB, Mentore JL, Moonseong H, et al. (1999). Antipsychotic-induced weight gain a comprehensive research synthesis. *American Journal of Psychiatry*, **156**: 1686–96.

American psychiatric Association (2000). *Diagnostic and statistical manual of mental disorders*, 4th ed., revised. American Psychiatric Association, Washington, DC.

Andreasen NC (1989). The Scale for the Assessment of Negative Symptoms (SANS): conceptual and theoretical foundations. *British Journal of Psychiatry*, **155**(suppl. 7): 49–58.

Andreasen NC (1995). Symptoms, signs and diagnosis of schizophrenia. *Lancet*, **346**: 477–81.

Andreasen NC, Carpenter WT, Kane JM, et al. (2005). Remission in schizophrenia: proposed criteria and rationale for consensus. *American Journal of Psychiatry*, **162**: 441–9.

Andreasson S, Allebeck P, Engstrom A, et al. (1987). Cannabis and schizophrenia. *Lancet*, **ii**: 1483–6.

Arsenault L, Cannon M, Witton J, Murray RM, et al. (2004a). Causal association between cannabis and psychosis: examination of the evidence. *British Journal of Psychiatry*, **184**: 110–17.

Arsenault L, Cannon M, Witton J, Murray RM, et al. (2004b). Cannabis as a potential causal factor in schizophrenia. In DJ Castle and RM Murray, eds. *Marijuana and Madness*, Cambridge University Press, Cambridge pp. 101–118.

Aylward E, Walker E, Bettes B (1984). Intelligence in schizophrenia: meta-analysis of the research. *Schizophrenia Bulletin*, **10**: 430–59.

Bell M, Bryson G, Greig T, et al. (2001). Neurocognitive enhancement therapy with work therapy. *Archives of General Psychiatry*, **58**: 763–8.

Berrios GE (1999). Classifications in psychiatry: a conceptual history. *Australian and New Zealand Journal of Psychiatry*, **33**: 145–60.

Bleuler E (1911). *Dementia Praecox order Gruppe Schizophrenien*. Deuticke, Leipzig.

Boydell J, van Os, J, Lambri M, et al. (2003). Incidence of schizophrenia in south-east London between 1965 and 1997. British Journal of Psychiatry, 182: 45–9.

Bradbury TN and Miller GA (1985). Season of birth in schizophrenia: a review of the evidence, methodology and etiology. Psychological Bulletin, 98: 569–94.

Buckley PF (1998). Substance abuse and schizophrenia: a review. Journal of Clinical Psychiatry, 59: 26–30.

Buckley PF (2007). Factors that influence treatment success in schizophrenia. Journal of Clinical psychiatry, 115: 93–100.

Buckley PF and Stahl SM (2007). Pharmacological treatment of negative symptoms of schizophrenia: therapeutic opportunity or cul de sac? Acta Psychiatrica Scandinavica, 115: 93–100.

Buckley PF, Noffsinger S, Smith DA, et al. (2003). Treatment of the psychotic patient who is violent. Psychiatric Clinics of North America, 26: 231–72.

Buckley PF, Wirshing DA, Bhushan P, et al. (2007). Lack of insight in schizophrenia: impact on treatment adherence. CNS Drugs, 21: 129–41.

Buckley PF (2008). Update on the etiology and treatment of schizophrenia and bipolar disorder. CNS Spectrums, (in press).

Buckley PF, Miller BJ, Foster A (2008). Schizophrenia and metabolic disturbances: host vulnerability and the risk of antipsychotic therapy. Focus, 6 (2): 172–9.

Buka SL, Tsuang MT, Torrey EF, et al. (2001). Maternal infections and subsequent psychosis among offspring. Archives of General Psychiatry, 58: 1032–7.

Bustillo J, Lauriello J, Horan W, et al. (2001). The psychosocial treatment of schizophrenia: an update. American Journal of Psychiatry, 158: 163–75.

Byrne M, Agerbo E, Ewald H, et al. (2003). Paternal age and risk of schizophrenia. Archives of General Psychiatry, 60: 673–8.

Cannon TD, Rosso IM, Hollister JM, et al. (2000). A prospective cohort study of genetic and perinatal influences in the etiology of schizophrenia. Schizophrenia Bulletin, 26: 351–66.

Carpenter WT (2001). Evidence-based treatment for first-episode schizophrenia? American Journal of Psychiatry, 158: 1771–3.

Carpenter WT Jr, Heinrichs WD, Alphs LD (1985). Treatment of negative symptoms. Schizophrenia Bulletin, 11: 440–52.

Castle DJ and Murray RM (1991). The neurodevelopmental basis of sex differences in schizophrenia. Psychological Medicine, 21: 565–75.

Castle DJ and Murray RM (1993). The epidemiology of late onset schizophrenia. Schizophrenia Bulletin, 19: 691–700.

Castle DJ, Abel K, Takei N, Murray Rm (1995). Gender differences in schizophrenia: hormonal effect, or subtypes? Schizophrenia Bulletin, 30: 274–8.

Castle DJ and Murray RM (eds) (2004). Marijuana and madness. Cambridge University Press, Cambridge.

Castle DJ, Trann N, Alderton D (2008). In DJ Castle, D Copolov, T Wykes, K Mueser, eds. *Pharmacological and psychosocial treatments for schizophrenia*, 2nd ed. pp. 1–22, Informa, London.

Conley RR and Kelly DL (2001). Management of treatment-resistant schizophrenia. *Biological Psychiatry*, **50**: 898–911.

Cooper JE, Kendell RE, Gurland BJ, *et al.* (1972). *Psychiatric diagnosis in New York and London*. Oxford: Oxford University Press, 1972.

Copolov D and Castle DJ (2007). In: Castle DJ, Copolov D, Wykes T, Mueser K, eds. *Pharmacological and psychosocial treatments for schizophrenia*, 2nd ed. Informa, London.

Correll CU, Leucht S, Kane JM (2004). Lower risk for tardive dyskinesia with second-generation antipsychotics: a systematic review of 1-year studies. *American Journal of Psychiatry*, **161**: 414–25.

Croudacre TJ, Kayne R, Jones PB, *et al.* (2000). Non-linear relationship between and index of social deprivation, psychiatric admission prevalence and the incidence of psychosis. *Psychological Medicine*, **30**: 177–85.

Crow TJ (1980). Positive and negative symptoms and the role of dopamine in schizophrenia. *British Journal of Psychiatry*, **346**: 383–6.

David AS, Malmberg A, Brandt L, *et al.* (1997). IQ and risk for schizophrenia: a population-based cohort study. *Psychological Medicine*, **27**: 1311–23.

Davidson L, Chinman M, Sells D, *et al.* (2006). Peer support among adults with mental illness: a report from the field. *Schizophrenia Bulletin*, **32**: 443–50.

Davis J, Chen N, Glick ID (2003). A meta-analysis of the efficacy of second-generation antipsychotics. *Archives of General Psychiatry*, **60**: 553–64.

Der G, Gupta S, Murray RM (1990). Is schizophrenia disappearing? *Lancet*, **335**: 51316.

Dixon L, Adams C, Lucksted A (2000). Update on the family psychoeducation of schizophrenia. *Schizophrenia Bulletin*, **26**: 21–46.

Done DJ, Johnstone EC, Frith CD, *et al.* (1991). Complications of pregnancy and delivery in relation to psychosis in adult life: data from the British perinatal mortality survey sample. *British Medical Journal*, **302**: 1576–80.

Drake RE and Mueser KT (2000). Psychosocial approaches to dual diagnosis. *Schizophrenia Bulletin*, **26**: 105–18.

Drake RE, Essock SM, Shaner A, *et al.* (2001). Implementing dual diagnosis services for clients with severe mental illness. *Psychiatric Services*, **52**: 469–76.

Druss BG, Rohrbaugh RM, Levinson CM, *et al.* (2001). Integrated medical care for patients with serious psychiatric illness. *Archives of General Psychiatry*, **28**: 861–8.

Elkis H (2007). Treatment resistant schizophrenia. *Psychiatric Clinics of North America*, **3**: 511–34.

Emsley R and Oosthuizen P (2004). Evidence-based pharmacotherapy of schizophrenia. *International Journal of Neurpsychopharmacology*, **7**: 219–38.

Faris R and Dunham HW (1960). *Mental disorders in urban areas*, 2nd ed. Hafner, New York.

Fenton W and McGlashan T (1986). The prognostic significance of obsessive-compulsive symptoms in schizophrenia. *American Journal of Psychiatry*, **143**: 437–41.

Fish B (1977). Neurobiological antecedents of schizophrenia in children. *Archives of General Psychiatry*, **34**: 1297–313.

Garety P, Fowler D, Kuipers E (2000). Cognitive-behavioural therapy for medication-resistant symptoms. *Schizophrenia Bulletin*, **43**: 71–90.

Geddes JR and Lawrie SM (1995). Obstetric complications and schizophrenia: a meta-analysis. *British Journal of Psychiatry*, **167**: 786–93.

Geddes J, Freemantle N, Harrison P, *et al.* (2000). Atypical antipsychotics in the treatment of schizophrenia: systematic overview and regression analysis. *British Medical Journal*, **321**: 1371–6.

Gilbert M, Miller K, Berk L, Ho V, Castle D (2003). The scope for psychosocial treatments for psychoaia: an overview of Collaborative Therapy. *Australasian Psychiatry*, **11**: 220–4.

Glatt SJ, Faraone SV, Tsuang MT (2003). Association between a functional catechol O-methyltransferase gene polymorphism and schizophrenia: meta-analysis of case-control and family-based studies. *American Journal of Psychiatry*, **160**: 469–76.

Goff DC and Freudenreich O (2004). Focus on polypharmacy in schizophrenia: does anyone truly benefit. International *Journal of Neuropsychopharmacology*, **7**: 109–11.

Gottesman II and Shields J (1982). *Schizophrenia: the epigenetic puzzle*. Cambridge University Press, Cambridge.

Gottesman II and Gould TD (2003). The endophenotype concept in psychiatry. *American Journal of Psychiatry*, **160**: 889–96.

Green AI, Canuso CM, Brenner MJ, *et al.* (2003). Detection and management of comorbidity in patients with schizophrenia. *Psychiatric Clinics of North America*, **26**: 115–39.

Green MF (1996). What are the functional consequences of neurocognitive deficits in schizophrenia? *American Journal of Psychiatry*, **153** (3): 321–30.

Hafner H, Maurer K, Loffler W, *et al.* (1993). The influence of age and sex on the onset and early course of schizophrenia. *British Journal of Psychiatry*, **162**: 80–6.

Halperin S, Nathan P, Drummond P, Castle D (2000). A cognitive-behavioural group based intervention for social anxiety in schizophrenia. *Australian and New Zealand Journal of Psychiatry*, **34**: 809–13.

Harrigan EP, Micelli JJ, AnzanioR, *et al.* (2004). A randomised evaluation of the effects of six antipsychotic agents on QTc, in the absence and presence of metabolic inhibition. *Journal of Clinical Psychopharmacology*, **24**: 62–9.

Harrison G, Owens D, Holton A, et al. (1988). A prospective study of sever mental disorder in Afro-Caribbean patients. *Psychological Medicine*, **182**: 45–9.

Harrison G, Hopper K, Craig T, et al. (2001). Recovery from psychotic illness: a 15- and 25-year international follow-up study. *British Journal of Psychiatry*, **178**: 506–17.

Harrison PJ and Weinberger DR (2005). Schizophrenia genes, gene expression and neuropathology: on the matter of their convergence. *Molecular Psychiatry*, **10**: 40–68.

Harvey PD and Cornblatt B (2008). Pharmacological treatment of cognition in schizophrenia: an idea whose time has come. *American Journal of Psychiatry*, **165**: 163–5.

Heaton RK, Baade LE, Johnstone KL (1978). Neuropsychological test results associated with psychotic disorders in adults. *Psychological Bulletin*, **85**: 141–62.

Henderson DC, Cagliero E, Gray C, et al. (2000). Clozapine, diabetes mellitus, weight gain and lipid abnormalities: a five year naturalistic study. *American Journal of Psychiatry*, **157**: 875–981.

Hoenig J (1983). The concept of schizophrenia: Kraepelin-Bleuler-Schneider. *British Journal of Psychiatry*, **142**: 547–56.

Hogarty G, Kornblith SJ, Greenwald D, et al. (1997). The year trial of personal therapy among schizophrenic patients living with or independent of family. *American Journal of Psychiatry*, **154**: 1504–13.

Huey LY, Lefley HP, Shern DL, et al. (2007). Families and schizophrenia: the view from advocacy. *Psychiatric Clinics of North America*, **30**: 549–66.

Jablensky A, Sartorius N, Ernberg G, et al. (1992). Schizophrenia: manifestation, incidence and course in different cultures. A World Health Organisation ten country study. Psychological Medicine Monograph 20.

Jablensky A, McGrath J, Herrman H, et al. (1999). National Study of Mental Health and Wellbeing. Report 4. People Living with Psychotic Illness: An Australian Study. Canberra: Commonwealth of Australia.

James W, Preston N, Koh G, et al. (2004). A group intervention that assists patients with dual diagnosis reduce their drug use: a randomised controlled trial. *Psychological Medicine*, **34**: 983–90.

Johnstone EC, Crow TJ, Frith CD, et al. (1976). Cerebral ventricular size and cognitive impairment in chronic schizophrenia. *Lancet*, **2**: 924–6.

Jones PB and Buckley PF (2006). *Schizophrenia*. Elsevier, London.

Jones P and Murray R (1991). The genetics of schizophrenia is the genetics of neurodevelopment. *British Journal of Psychiatry*, **158**: 615–23.

Jones P, Rogers B, Murray R, et al. (1994). Child development risk factors for adult schizophrenia in the British 1946 birth cohort. *Lancet*, **334**: 1398–402.

Kane J, Honigfeld G, Singer J, et al. (1988). Clozapine for the treatment-resistant schizophrenic: a randomised comparison with chlorpromazine. *Archives of General Psychiatry*, **45**: 789–96.

Kapur S and Remmington G (2001). Dopamine D2 receptors and their role in atypical antipsychotic action: still necessary but not sufficient. *Biological psychiatry*, **50**: 873–83.

Keefe RSE, Silva SG, Perkins DO, *et al.* (1999). The effects of atypical antipsychotic drugs on neurocognitive impairment in schizophrenia: a review and meta-analysis. *Schizophrenia Bulletin*, **25**: 201–22.

Kendler KS, McGuire M, Gruemberg AM, *et al.* (1993). The Roscommon family study. III. Schizophrenia-related personality disorders in relatives. *Archives of General Psychiatry*, **50**: 781–8.

Kessler RC, McGonagle KA, Zhao S, *et al.* (1994). Lifetime and 12-month prevalence of DSM-III-R psychiatric disorders in the United States: results from the National Comorbidity Survey. *Archives of General Psychiatry*, **52**: 8–19.

Keuneman R, Weerasundera R, Castle D (2002). The role of ECT in schizophrenia. *Australasian Psychiatry*, **10**: 385–8.

Khashan AS, Abel KM, McNamee R, *et al.* (2008). Higher risk of offspring with schizophrenia following antenatal exposure to sever adverse life events. *Archives of General Psychiatry*, **65**: 146–52.

Kingsep P, Nathan P, Castle D (2003). Cognitive behavioural group treatment for social anxiety in schizophrenia. *Schizophrenia Research*, **63**: 121–9.

Kirkpatrick B, Buchanan RW, McKenney PD, *et al.* (1989). The Schedule for the Assessment of the Deficit Syndrome: an instrument for research in schizophrenia. *Psychiatry Research*, **30**: 119–23.

Kraepelin E (1896). *Psychiatrie*, 5th ed. Barth, Leipzig.

Lacro JP, Dunn LB, Dolder CR, *et al.* (2002). Prevalence of and risk factors for medication non-adherence in patients with schizophrenia. *Journal of Clinical Psychiatry*, **63**: 892–909.

Lauriello J, Bustillo J, Ketih SJ (1999). A critical review of research on psychosocial treatment of schizophrenia. *Biological Psychiatry*, **46**: 1409–17.

Lehman AF (1999). Developing an outcomes-oriented approach for the treatment of schizophrenia. *Journal of Clinical Psychiatry*, **60**: 30–5.

Lehman T Lieberman JA, Perkins DO, *et al.* (2004). Treatment guidelines for the management of patients with schizophrenia, second edition. *American Journal of Psychiatry*, **161**: 1–56.

Leff J and Vaughan C (1985). *Expressed emotion in families: its significance for mental illness.* Guildford, New York.

Lewis G, David A, Andreasson S, *et al.* (1992). Schizophrenia and city life. *Lancet*, **340**: 137–40.

Leucht S, Barnes TR, Kissling W, *et al.* (2003). Relapse prevention in schizophrenia with new-generation antipsychotics: a systematic review and exploratory meta-analysis of randomized, controlled trials. *American Journal of Psychiatry*, **160**: 1209–22.

Lieberman JA, Perkins D, Belger A, *et al.* (2001). The early stages of schizophrenia: speculation on the pathogenesis, pathophysiology, and therapeutic approaches. *Biological Psychiatry*, **50**: 884–97.

Lieberman JA, Stroup TS, McEvoy JP, et al. (2005). Effectiveness of anti-psychotic drugs in patients with chronic schizophrenia. *New England Journal of medicine*, **353**: 1209–23.

Lieberman J, Stoup S, Perkins DO (2006). *Textbook of schizophrenia*. American Psychiatric Press, Washington DC.

Liddle PF, Friston KJ, Frith CD, et al. (1992). Patterns of cereberal blood flow in schizophrenia. *British Journal of Psychiatry*, **160**: 179–86.

Liddle P, Carpenter WT, Crow T (1994). Syndromes of schizophrenia. *British Journal of Psychiatry*, **165**: 721–7.

Leonhard K (1979). *The classification of endogenous psychoses*, 5th ed. (translated R Berman) Irvington Publishers, New York.

Lubman DI and Sundram S (2003). Substance misuse in patients with schizophrenia: a primary care guide. *Medical Journal of Australia*, **178**: S71–S75.

Marder SR, Essock SM, Miller AL, et al. (2004). Physical health monitoring of patients with schizophrenia. *American Journal of Psychiatry*, **161**: 1334–49.

Masellis M, Basile V, Ozdemir V, et al. (2000). Pharmacogenetics of anti-psychotic treatment: lessons learned from clozapine. *Biological Psychiatry*, **47**: 252–66.

McClellan M, Susser E, King M (2007). Schizophrenia: a common disease caused by multiple rare alleles. *British Journal of Psychiatry*, **191**: 190–4.

McEvoy JP, Lieberman JA, Stroup TS, et al. (2006). Effectiveness of clozapine versus olanzapine, quetiapine, and risperidone in patients with schizophrenia who did not respond to prior atypical antpsychotic treatment. *American Journal of Psychiatry*, **163**: 600–10.

McGlashan T and Carpenter W (1976). Postpsychotic depression in schizophrenia. *Archives of General Psychiatry*, **33**: 231–9.

McGlashan TH, Miller TJ, Woods SW (2001). Pre-onset detection and intervention research in schizophrenia psychoses: current estimates of benefit and risks. *Schizophrenia Bulletin*, **27**: 563–70.

McGorry PD (2002). The recognition and optimal management of early psychosis: an evidence-based reform. *World Psychiatry*, **1**: 76–83.

McGrath JJ and Murray RM (2003). Risk factors for schizophrenia: from conception to birth. In SR Hirsch and DR Weinberger, eds. *Schizophrenia*, pp. 163–83. Blackwell, Oxford.

McGuire PK and Frith CD (1996). Disordered functional connectivity in schizophrenia. *Psychological Medicine*, **26**: 663–7.

Mednick SA, Machon RA, Huttunen MO, et al. (1988). Adult schizophrenia following prenatal exposure to an influenza epidemic. *Archives of General Psychiatry*, **45**: 171–6.

Meltzer HY, Alphs L, Green AI, et al. (2003). Clozapine treatment for suicidality in schizophrenia. International Suicide Prevention Trial (InterSePT). *Archives of General Psychiatry*, **60**: 82–91.

Meyer JM (2003). Cardiovascular illness and hyperlipidemia in patients with schizophrenia. In JM Meyer and Nasrallah HA, eds. pp. 53–80. American Psychiatric Publishing, Washington, DC.

Mortensen PB, Pederson CB, Westergaard T, *et al.* (1999). Effects of family history and place and season of birth on the risk of schizophrenia. *New England Journal of Medicine*, **340**: 603–8.

Murdoch D, Keating GM (2006). Sertindole: A review of its use in schizophrenia. *CNS Drugs*, **20**: 233–55.

Murray RM (1994). Neurodevelopmental schizophrenia: the rediscovery of dementia praecox. *British Journal of Psychiatry*, **165**: 6–12.

Murray RM, Lewis SW, Reveley AM (1985). Towards and aetiological classification of schizophrenia. *Lancet*, **1**: 1023–6.

Murray RM, O'Callaghan E, Castle DJ, Lewis SW (1992). A neurodevelopmental approach to the classification of schizophrenia. *Schizophrenia Bulletin*, **18**: 319–32.

Newcomer J (2007). Antipsychotic medications: metabolic and cardiovascular risk. *Journal of Clinical Psychiatry*, **68**(suppl. 4): 813.

O'Callaghan E, Sham P, Takei N, *et al.* (1991). Schizophrenia after prenatal exposure to the 1957 A2 influenza epidemic. *Lancet*, **337**: 1248–50.

Pantelis C, Velakoulis D, McGorry PD (2003). Neuroanatomical abnormalities before and after onset of psychosis. *Lancet*, **361**: 281–8.

Patil ST, Jhnang, Martenyi F, *et al.* (2007). Activation of mglu2/3 receptors as a new therapeutic approach to treat schizophrenia: a randomised phase 2 clinical trial. *Nature Medicine*, **13**: 1102–7.

Pearlson GD and Calhoun V (2007). Structural and functional imaging in psychiatric disorders. *Canadian Journal of Psychiatry*, **52**: 158–66.

Petronis A and Kennedy JL (1995). Unstable genes, unstable mind. *American Journal of Psychiatry*, **152**: 164–72.

Pokos V and Castle DJ (2006). Prevalence of comorbid anxiety disorders in schizophrenioa spectrum disorders: a literature review. *Current Psychiatry Reviews*, **2**: 285–307.

Poulton R, Caspi A, Moffett TE, *et al.* (2000). Children's self reported psychotic symptoms and adult schizophreniform disorder: a 15-year longitudinal study. *Archives of General Psychiatry*, **57**: 1053–8.

Robinson DG, Woerner MG, McMeniman M, *et al.* (2004). Symptomatic and functional recovery from a first episode of schizophrenia or schizoaffective disorder. *American Journal of Psychiatry*, **161**: 473–9.

Russell AJ, Munro JC, Jones PB, *et al.* (1997). Schizophrenia and the myth of intellectual decline. *American Journal of Psychiatry*, **154**: 635–9.

Schneider K (1959). *Clinical psychopathology*. Translated by HW Hamilton. Grune and Stratton, New York.

Schulz SC, Barnes T, Buckley PF (2003). Treatment resistant schizo-phrenia. In SR Hirsch and DR Weinberger, eds. *Schizophrenia*, pp. 486–8 Blackwell, Oxford.

Selten JP and Sijben N (1994). First admission rate for schizophrenia in immigrants to The Netherlands: the Dutch National Register. *Social Psychiatry and Psychiatric Epidemiology*, **29**: 71–2.

Sharma T and Antonova L (2003). Cognitive function in schizophrenia: deficits, functional consequences, and future treatment. *Psychiatric Clinics of North America*, **26**: 25–40.

Simmons S, Coid J, Joseph P, *et al*. (2001). Community mental health team management in severe mental illness: a systematic review. *British Journal of Psychiatry*, **178**: 497–502.

Siris S (2000). Depression in schizophrenia: perspective in the era of atypical antipsychotic agents. *American Journal of Psychiatry*, **157**: 1379–89.

Sudath RL, Christison GW, Torrey EF, *et al*. (1990). Anatomical abnormalities in the brains of monozygotic twins discordant for schizophrenia. *New England Journal of Medicine*, **322**: 789–94.

Susser E and Lin P (1992). Schizophrenia after prenatal exposure to the Dutch hunger winter of 1944-1945. *Archives of General Psychiatry*, **49**: 983–8.

Torrey EF and Miller J (2002). *The invisible plague. The rise of mental illness from 1750 to the present.* Rutgers University Press, New Jersey.

Troy M, Buchanan B, Buckley P, *et al*. (2007). The Texas Medication Algorithm Project antipsychotic algorithm for schizophrenia: 2006 Update. *Journal of Clinical Psychiatry*, **68** (11): 1751–62.

VanOs J, Castle DJ, Takei N, *et al*. (1996). Psychotic illness in ethnic minorities: clarification form the 1991 census. *Psychological Medicine*, **26**: 203–8.

Verdoux H, Castle DJ, Murray RM (2005). Cannabis and psychosis proneness. In *Marijuana and madness*, pp. 75–88. Cambridge University Press, Cambridge.

Walker E and Lewine RJ (1994). Predication of adult-onset schizophrenia from childhood home movies of the patients. *American Journal of Psychiatry*, **147**: 1052–6.

Walsh E, Buchanan A, Fahy T (2002). Violence and schizophrenia: examining the evidence. *British Journal of Psychiatry*, **180**: 490–5.

Waddington JL and O'Callaghan E (1997). What makes an antipsychotic 'atypical'? Conserving the definition. *CNS Drugs*, **7**: 341–6.

Wallbeck K, Cheine M, Essali A, Adams C (1999). Evidence for clozapine's effectiveness in schizophrenia: a systematic review and meta-analysis of randomized trials. *American Journal of Psychiatry*, **156**: 990–9.

Watt NF (1978). Patterns of childhood social development in adult schizophrenics. *Archives of General Psychiatry*, **35**: 160–5.

Weiden PJ and Buckley PF (2007). Switching antipsychotic medications. *Journal of Clinical Psychiatry*, **68** (suppl. 6) 14–23.

Weiden PJ and Casey DE (1999). 'Polypharmacy': combining antipsychotic medications in the treatment of schizophrenia. *Journal of Practical Psychiatry and Behavioral Health*, **5**: 229–33.

Weiden PJ, Buckley PF, Grody M (2007). Understanding and treating first episode schizophrenia. *Psychiatric Clinics of North America*, **30**: 481–511.

Weinberger DR (1995). Schizophrenia: from neuropathology to neuro-development. *Lancet*, **346**: 552–7.

Weinberger DR, Egan MF, Bertolini A, *et al.* (2001). Prefrontal neurons and the genetics of schizophrenia. *Biological Psychiatry*, **50**: 825–44.

Wessley S, Castle D, Der G, *et al.* (1991). Schizophrenia and Afro-Caribbeans. A case-control study. *British journal of Psychiatry*, **159**: 795–801.

World Health Organisation (1993). *The ICD-10 classification of mental and behavioural disorders: diagnostic criteria for research*. World Health Organisation, Geneva.

Wright IC, Rabe-Hesketh S, Woodruff PW, *et al.* (2000). Meta-analysis of regional brain volumes in schizophrenia. *American Journal of Psychiatry*, **157**: 16–25.

Wykes T and Castle D (2007). Cognition In DJ Castle, D Copolov, T Wykes, K Mueser, eds. *Pharmacological and psychosocial treatments for schizophrenia*, 2nd ed. Informa, London.

Zubin J and Spring B (1977). Vulnerability—a new view of schizophrenia. *Journal of Abnormal Psychology*, **86**: 103–26.

Index

125

running commentary
  hallucinations 4t

S

SAD see social anxiety
  disorder (SAD)
Scale for the Assessment of
  Negative Symptoms
  (SANS) 16
Scale for the Assessment of
  Positive Symptoms
  (SAPS) 16–17
Schedule for the Deficit
  Syndrome (SDS) 18–19
schizo-obsessive disorder 26
schizoaffective disorder 5b, 8
schizophrenia construct,
  historical antecedents
  of 4–7
schizophreniform
  psychosis 7
schizotypal personality
  disorder (SPD) 8, 39
Schneider, K. 5b, 6–7
Schooler, N. 92
season of birth, and
  schizophrenia 39–40
selective serotonin reuptake
  inhibitors (SSRIs) 26,
  103, 106
self-medication 27
sensory gating abnormalities
  49–50
serotonergic mechanisms
  26, 53, 76
serotonin 5HT-2A
  receptors 53
serotonin noradrenaline
  reuptake inhibitors
  (SNRIs) 103, 106
sertindole 53, 67, 105, 108
sertraline 106
sexual dysfunction 67, 69b,
  90, 103
Shields, J. 38
sibutramine 84
side effects
  medications for 104, 107
  see also antipsychotics;
    clozapine
silly hebephrenia 9
simple schizophrenias 10b
Singer Wynne 43
single photon emission
  tomography (SPECT) 48
sluggish catatonia 9
smoking
  and clozapine 111
  risks of 84

SNRIs see serotonin nora-
  drenaline reuptake inhibitors (SNRIs)
social anxiety disorder
  (SAD) 24, 25, 80, 81b
social skills training 74–5,
  80–1
sodium valproate 29, 72,
  104, 107, 114
SSRIs see selective serotonin
  reuptake inhibitors
  (SSRIs)
static encephalopathy 46
Stengel 26
strengths model, of care
  57–8
substance use disorder (SUD)
  first episode psychosis
    (FEP) 90–1
  impact of 27, 28b
  medication adherence,
    problem of 85
  and mental health,
    integrated programmes
    for 85–6
  and outcomes 34
  versus primary psychotic
    disorders 26–7
subtypes, of schizophrenia
  8–11
  DSM-ICD classification 10
  Leonhard's classification
    8, 9
SUD see substance use
  disorder (SUD)
Sudath, R.L. 38
suicide, and depression
  24–5
Sundram, S. 27b
symptoms, of schizophrenia
  DMM-1V R critieria 4t, 7
  first rank (Schneider) 6
  ICD-10 criteria 4t
  onset of 7
  positive psychotic
    symptoms 6
  primary and secondary
    (Bleuler) 5–6, 5b
syphilis 5
Szasz, T. 3
Szasz, Thomas 3

T

tardive dyskinesia (TD) 62,
  65–5
TCAs see tricyclic
  antidepressants (TCAs)
temazepam 107
thioridazine 105, 108

third person conversing 4t
thioridazine 67
thought broadcast 4t, 6b
thought echo 4t
thought insertion 4t
thought withdrawal 4t, 6b
TMS (transcranial magnetic
  stimulation), use of 77
topiramate 74, 84, 107
tricyclic antidepressants
  (TCAs) 103, 105
trifluoperazine 105, 108
trimipramine 105

U

undifferentiated
  schizophrenias 10b
US-UK diagnostic project
  31–2

V

valproate 73
valproic acid 94
varenicline 84
venlafaxine 106
ventricular brain ratio
  (VBR) 46
violent behaviour see
  behavioural disturbance,
  acute
voluble catatonia 9

W

weight gain 28–9, 67, 69b,
  72, 73, 84, 102, 109, 112
Weinberger, D. 50
white blood cell count
  (WBC) 70, 72b
women, with schizophrenia
  childbirth 89–90
  menstrual cycle, and oes-
    tregen flux 90
  see also pregnancy
workforce, helping people
  into
  supported employment
    programmes 75, 86–7
  work, barriers to obtaining
    36
  workplace-level
    interventions 87

Z

ziprasidone 29, 48, 53, 64t,
  67, 73, 105, 108
zuclopenthixol 83, 105, 108